Testimonials

From Middle School Students

"A couple months ago, while speaking at a middle school in Oregon, I was approached by a student who shared with me that my talk encouraged and inspired her to put forth the effort required to achieve her goals. She stated that she was committed to being a standout on her track team, improving her grades and being an overall better person!"

—**Zoe**

"Thank you for sharing your time and experience with me. It was meaningful and changed my perspective to hear about what happened in high school. My favorite part was when you started talking to people and making friends because it moved me." Eli
"You inspired me to achieve my goals!"

—**Judith**

"My favorite part was that you believed in yourself, because I have a hard time believing in myself in hard situations."

—**Amara**

"Thank you for sharing your story. It was very inspiring! I hope you inspire more people with your experience."

Other Testimonials

"Bill's story is one that needs to be heard. To truly put you in another person's shoes is one thing, but to hear Bill speak about the challenges he faced and the feelings he felt throughout his endeavor is revealing. It inspires others to be better people, whether it's you who needs the encouragement to stand up for yourself or if you can be the champion to help another succeed. It's with this true passion that Bill Deering inspires others to more with what they have."

—**Berto Cerrillo, Director of Student Life and Leadership, Portland Community College.**

"Input on program evaluations overwhelming confirmed that your presentation increased awareness about bullying and biases against people with disabilities. I personally found your message to be passionate and heartening. I am also amazed by the way you have overcome the speech difficulties that once created such a barrier for you. Your courage has touched the lives of many."

—Debbie Richards, Co-Chair, Special Assistant to the
President, West Virginia University @ Parkersburg

"Mr. Deering's presentation helped to empower these students to share their experiences with him and the rest of their class-mates. As the program concluded and the students were dismissed many students came to the front of the auditorium; I assumed to speak to Mr. Deering. Actually, students just wanted to shake his hand. In my 20 years of education, it is the first time that I have seen students connect this way with a speaker."

—Kristi Greene, Assistant Principal,
Halstead Middle School

I HAVE SOMETHING TO SAY

A Memoir About Stuttering, Bullies, and Kindness

Publishing Mentor: Kate Butler Books

Cover and Interior Design by Melissa Williams Design
mwbookdesign.com

Artwork by Anthony Van Bruggen
All photographs are courtesy of the author.

Copyedting by Heather Shafter and Ariane Lewis

I HAVE SOMETHING TO SAY

A Memoir About Stuttering, Bullies, and Kindness

William J. Deering

To anyone who has ever felt the sting from bullying and to those who struggle to fit in, I stand with you. This book is dedicated to you.

And to the brave souls willing to extend kindness when it is not the popular thing to do, thank you. This book is dedicated to you as well.

I hope my personal story will help others understand what a difference a simple kind gesture or the impact a few positive words can make to a person whose life struggle separates him from the crowd.

To my family, friends, and classmates, I also dedicate this book to you with gratitude.

Contents

List of Illustrations

Foreword

As a middle-school principal, I knew when I met Bill that I had to have him speak at my school. And I was right. His story described a challenging, often painful, and triumphant journey that people from all walks of life can appreciate.

Bill's empowering and inspirational presentation focused on how he overcame challenges he encountered due to a severe stuttering disability. His words deeply resonated with my students and staff. Bill's testimony was detailed, heartfelt, and inspirational. It dealt with the negative effects of bullying, managing adversity, breaking through barriers of ignorance, and the importance of working as a team to reach excellence. He demonstrated to all of us that people with various abilities can work through their personal limitations.

Bill's life experience and testimony has reaffirmed my own personal belief that all of us must be committed to creating a school environment in which children feel safe, secure, and loved. As the father of a daughter with special needs, I felt an immediate connection with Bill. I believe each of us must do whatever it takes to help every child, without exception, lead productive, enjoyable, and meaningful lives. During my thirty-six years of experience as a teacher, administrator, and now a parent, I can state without reservation that Mr. Bill Deering has an incredible story to tell us about his remarkable life!

This book is sure to inspire students, parents, teachers, and administrators to embrace their individual limitations and adversities in a positive manner.

Gene C. McGorry, M.Ed., Ed.D.
Principal, Hamburg Area Middle School

Preface

I never thought I could write a book. As a kid, I struggled with writing. In high school, I avoided writing essays as much as I could.

When I got to community college, I had no choice but to write. I remember it would take me hours just to get a paragraph down. I never got above a C in any of my English classes, and I was so happy when they were over. But, somehow, I found a way to write this book. The truth is I wanted to put my story on paper more than I wanted not to write. I wanted to share my story with you.

During the writing of this book, I had a chance to relive my childhood experiences. I felt the anger, frustration, and sadness I felt growing up, which forced me to look at myself in a different way. As a second grader, I was not a fun person to be around when kids bullied me. I got my frustrations out by hitting them with my fists. I realize now that I, too, was a bully. I was angry and frustrated and wanted my victims to feel the pain I went through. And it wasn't okay. None of it, not what I went through and not what I put others through.

This book is for anyone who has ever been the victim of a bully. It's for anyone who's ever become a bully because of being a victim. Each of us has a choice to make. We can either become the thing we hate or rise above it. What does it look like to stand our ground in the face of conflict? What happens when we treat people the way we want to be treated? In the chapters that follow, I ask you to come with me on my journey from victim to bully to success. I figure if I can do it, why not you?

1

Using My Fists

Picture for a moment a six-year-old boy who is both excited and eager to enter first grade only to be laughed at by the other children. And he has no idea why. Now, imagine this boy is someone you know—your son, your brother, your friend, your student, or even you at that age. He looks like any other first-grader. True, he is big for his age. At four feet, six inches tall and eighty-five pounds, he is about forty pounds heavier than the average student. He may tower over everyone but otherwise he is physically normal in every respect. So, why the ridicule? And what can he do to make it stop?

At Independence Elementary School, I was that boy, and it didn't take long for me to figure out the role I was to play there. I was the kid the other kids bullied. I realized what made me stick out so much; I stuttered severely and people couldn't understand me. At the beginning of each class, my teacher took attendance, and when she called out my name, I said, "um-um-um-um-um-um-um-um-um-um-here." I stood apart from my classmates, but for the wrong reason. Every time I opened my mouth and stuttered, someone in class laughed at me. I learned early on that people looked at me differently because of my stutter. Instead of trying to help or acknowledge my stutter, kids laughed and my teacher overlooked it.

I couldn't understand why she never did anything about it, and never could gather the courage to ask her. I would have liked for her to make an effort to know me, to take me aside and ask, "Bill, what is it like for you when you stutter? I have no idea. Can you please tell me? I really want to know how I can support you through first grade so it's a great experience rather than one you want to avoid. How can I help?"

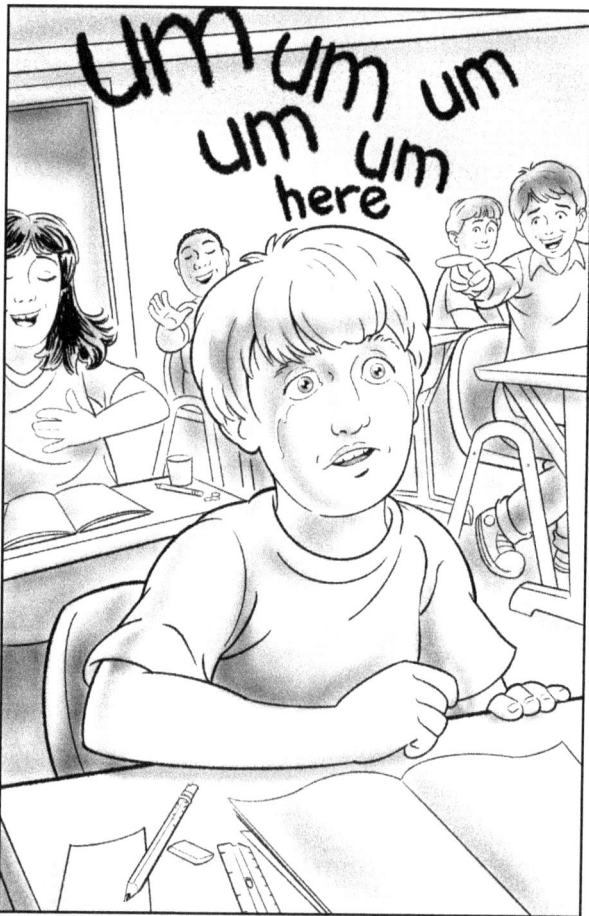

If she had said that, I would have answered, "Teach a lesson or maybe even dedicate a whole day to what it means to have tolerance, acceptance, and love for each other." Of course, I would not have known to say that at the time. I was trying to fit in and be accepted like all the other kids, and was just starting to figure out what separated me from them.

Having a conversation about the possibility for all first-graders to be eager and ready to learn regardless of their challenges, physical or otherwise—*that* would have made a difference. A group of teachers willing to take a stand for that lesson would have given me and many other students a very different experience in school. We would have been excited to come to class. The teachers would have been thrilled to have students willing and able to focus on learning. Kids on the playground would have been accepting of each other. Fighting could have been replaced with laughter, kindness, and joy. Instead, my elementary years were a very difficult part of my life.

Initially, I didn't even know what stuttering was. I thought to myself, "Why do *I* have to stick out? Why am *I* the only person in my class that does this? Why do *I* have to struggle so much just to get out one word? What's going on?"

My parents were notified of my challenges in school. The school counselor suggested I go to speech therapy, and my parents told me it would help. I listened because I knew they had my best interests in mind. I went to three thirty-minute sessions every week. At the time, almost every sound of the alphabet was difficult for me to say; there wasn't just one sound to work on. My therapist started by helping me with the sounds made by letters *b* and *d*. I found these to be the most difficult. Since they were my initials, saying my name was most challenging. My therapist gave me several techniques to use. One of them was to breathe before I spoke. This rarely worked for me.

I was easily angered because of the frustration stuttering

caused me. During recess, I took my frustrations out on the other kids on the playground, fighting anyone and everyone who laughed at me. If a kid made fun of me, I would punch or push him. I didn't really think about the consequences or how I was harming others. I didn't care. I lost my temper nearly every day. I found out quickly that using my fists to get kids to stop laughing at me wasn't looked upon fondly by my teacher or the principal, but I didn't know what else to do. I spent more time in the principal's office than any other kid in school. When I wasn't there, I was in class keeping to myself and only answering questions when called upon. But inside, I didn't want it to be that way. I just wanted to be a normal kid. I wanted people to get to know me before they decided whether they liked me. However, the hard truth was that it wasn't happening. Since I couldn't change the world, I changed myself. I adapted. Every time I punched someone who ridiculed me, I felt both satisfied and disappointed at the same time.

Luckily, my home life was pretty good. I lived in a neighborhood full of many kids my age and a few years older. For some reason, none of the neighborhood kids ever made fun of me. During the week, I did my homework and on weekends I played with my friends who lived near me. My parents still worried about me, though. My mom stuttered as a kid but outgrew it. As a result, she worried more than my dad did. He was frustrated that I couldn't say my words as well as my brothers, but didn't have enough patience to try to help me. I fought hard to control my stuttering around my dad because I didn't want him to yell at me. He was very stern so I often felt uncomfortable around him.

After a month or two of school, I finally made a few friends. One of them was Rick Roberts. He and I rode the school bus together and were in the same class. He was an African-American boy with a mini Afro. I was at least six inches taller than him. On most days, we ate lunch together. No matter how badly I stuttered, he never laughed at me. Even at the age of seven that fact was a bit surprising for me. Rick and I played kickball during recess. If anyone tried to make fun of me, he was there to defend me. This was a big relief because I no longer had to use my fists to get my point across; I didn't feel alone anymore. I had someone who was willing to be there for me as a friend. At that age, it meant a lot.

2

A Unique Skill

By second grade, I had grown another four inches and put on another twenty pounds. At four feet, ten inches and one-hundred-and-five pounds, I was at least six inches taller than the next kid in my grade. That didn't stop some of the kids from laughing at me, though. It was like they wanted to see what they could get away with before I beat them up. I still did that—especially when my classmates got me really mad by making fun of my stutter. I pushed, punched, or threatened to beat them up if they continued to tease me. This strategy worked until one of the kids reported my behavior to my teacher or the principal. It didn't take long before I knew the principal much better than I would have liked. I was deemed a troublemaker even though it was the other kids that always made fun of me. I couldn't help that I was much bigger than the other kids, and I had no problem taking my anger and frustration out on them at recess.

I began to fear using the school bathrooms because, as with every school, they are out of the teacher's sight and therefore the best place for bullies to harass their victims. Every day I became increasingly uncomfortable because I waited until I got home before going to the bathroom. Sometimes I would be in there for minutes at a time letting all of the urine out. I thought I was being tough. There were times when the pressure got so excruciating I wanted to give in and use the public bathroom, but I didn't. One afternoon I sat in math class toward the end of the day. I really had to go to the bathroom, but again stubbornly refused. When I realized I couldn't hold it any longer, I got up out of my seat and tried to walk to the door. Before I knew it, pee began running down my legs and all over the floor. My teacher was shocked. She put down newspaper to stop it from going everywhere. All of my classmates laughed. When I got home that day, I told my mom what happened. She was shocked to hear I had been holding it in every day and urged me to use the school bathroom in the future. From that point on, I did.

I was still going to speech therapy twice a week, but it was very frustrating. For those thirty minutes, my stutter seemed to be less severe. I even improved from session to session. But when I had to practice using the techniques I learned in public, nothing ever worked. My stuttering actually seemed to get worse. There were many times at home when I wanted to cry. I just wanted to stop stuttering and didn't understand why I couldn't. I felt if I didn't stutter my fellow students wouldn't have anything to laugh at me about. I felt like the school's laughingstock. As far as I knew, I was the only person in that entire school who stuttered.

In second grade, when I was eight, I developed a unique skill. I learned how to add, subtract, multiply, and divide numbers in my head. I loved collecting baseball cards. While my brothers and neighborhood friends played outside, I played my own games with the cards. One of them was adding up all of the home runs for a particular year from the statistics on the backsides of the cards. It didn't take me long before I could also subtract, multiply, and divide the numbers in my head. I became an instant wiz in my math class. I got to stick out in a good way for once! I really liked being the wiz kid.

My classmates and teacher were very impressed. My ability in arithmetic gave me the chance to be a regular kid instead of the tall, goofy kid who stuttered. Being able to shine in math class caused my classmates to see I actually had a brain. I was happier so my behavior improved. My classmates also saw that I wasn't just about beating people up, that I had a heart and could treat others the way I wanted to be treated.

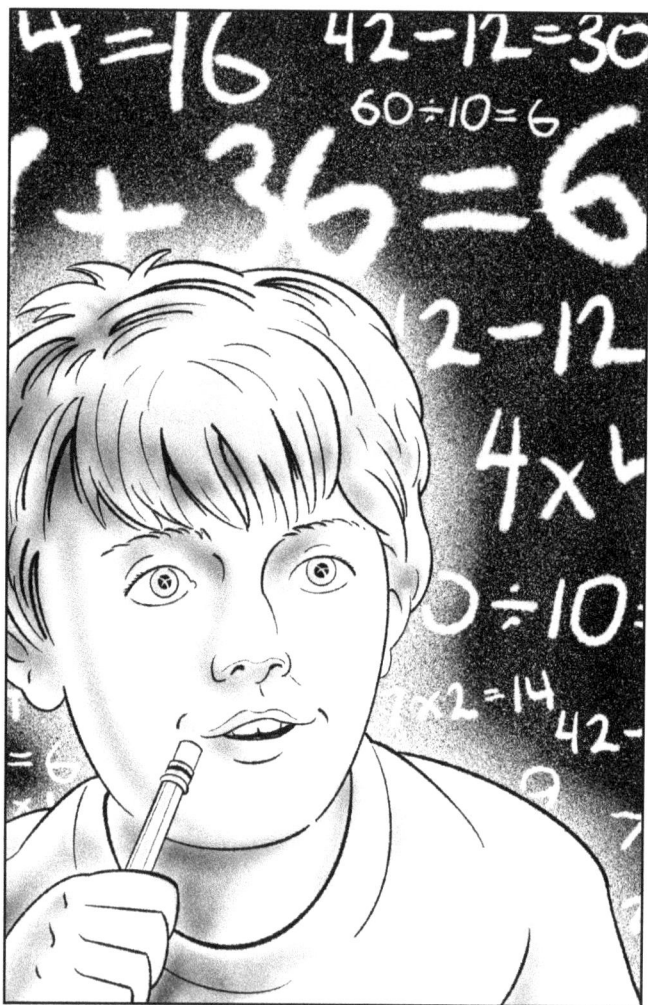

At the end of second grade, my parents told me I would be attending a special school in a nearby township. I was upset because I was just starting to fit in with my classmates. I didn't want to go. Some of my neighborhood friends weren't happy about it either because we attended elementary school together. My parents told me going to this school would help me with my temper. It became official during the summer of 1976.

When school started that September, I had to take a separate bus that picked me up right outside of my house. It was a small yellow van. While this was going on, the teachers at my old elementary school were on strike, which meant my neighborhood friends didn't have to go to school. The first day the yellow van picked me up, they were there to see me off. Now I really stuck out. I was not happy about it. I didn't want to go to this "special school," but I went anyway. When I arrived, I went into a classroom where there were ten other students. There were also two teachers in the front. Mrs. Goodall was the lead teacher. She was a thin woman with very light, grayish-brown hair that almost looked like an Afro. She was just over five feet tall. The other teacher was Mrs. O'Keefe. Mrs. O'Keefe was a little bit taller and heavyset with short, black hair. When I first saw them, I thought to myself, "They're not much taller than me. I wonder what I can get away with." By third grade, I was five feet tall and weighed one-hundred-and-twenty pounds. I was the tallest in my class again.

I looked around the room at the other students and thought to myself, "Why are they here? What is wrong with them? Do they have anger issues like me, or are they here for other reasons?" I couldn't figure them out. I was very cautious and didn't say much to anyone. I wanted to feel my classmates out before I opened myself up to them. We had recess and there was a playground, but I didn't want to play with anyone. I really didn't like being in a separate school from my friends at Independence Elementary.

A few days a week our class had physical education. Our

teacher for gym class was Mr. Richardson. He was a very ener-
getic guy. He really pushed us to work together as a team, but
many of my classmates—including me—didn't want any part
of that. We did our own thing. Each day went from 8:00 a.m.
to 2:30 p.m. I was so happy when I could get back on the little,
yellow van and go home for the day.

My neighborhood friends repeatedly asked me, "Bill,
what's it like? Do you like it? Why do you go there? Why
aren't you going to school with me?" I didn't know what to
say to all of those questions, so I just told them what I knew. I
said, "I don't really like it at all. I miss being with you and my
other friends. I go there to work on my bad temper." At least
that is what I thought at the time. I found out later that I was
there due to a learning disability.

When I wasn't at school, I played basketball in the local
recreational league during the late fall and winter months. It
was my first year playing in the league so I didn't know what
to expect. I was still stuttering severely, but when I got on the
basketball court with my team, stuttering didn't matter. What
mattered was winning our games and having fun. I usually
started on my team, mainly because I was at least four inches
taller than everyone else. I was in the recreational league for
kids aged nine to ten. There was another league for kids up
to age fifteen. I didn't score many points, but I hustled up
and down the court. My coach really appreciated how hard I
worked even though I scored a grand total of only four points
for the entire year.

All of our games were on Saturday. During my first year,
the team's record was four wins and six losses. I enjoyed
playing and being a part of a team because I knew that for
at least two hours a week, my teammates and people in the
league weren't going to make fun of my stutter.

After basketball season was over, I went back to hanging
out with my friends in the neighborhood. I had four friends I
enjoyed being around. Their names were Chet, Bob, Charlie,

and Peter. Peter was at my house a lot. He especially loved to come over when he knew my mom had gone grocery shopping. His parents were not around much, so he was at my house every Friday to help my mom unload the groceries, and then help eat them. Peter also friends with my brothers. He annoyed my dad a lot by calling every Saturday morning at 6 a.m. to ask if my brothers, Jonathan and Jamie, and I were ready to come out and play. I got to see Bob, Chet, and Charlie frequently as well. We played kickball, football, basketball, and baseball together. We also played board games, had sleepovers, or just hung out at each other's houses for dinner.

Third grade was almost over, and I was happy to hear that our class was moving to Independence Elementary School for fourth grade. Over the year, I had gotten to know my classmates. I liked some of them more than others. Both of my teachers were coming with us. I was not very happy about that. I didn't really like Mrs. Goodall. She was tough and pushed me. Mrs. O'Keefe challenged me, too, but seemed to be more caring and loving. When I shared with my neighborhood friends that I was returning to Independence Elementary School, they were ecstatic. My friend Rick Roberts was also happy to hear that. I saw him from time to time over my third-grade year.

Everyone said it must be nice for me to get back to normal, but I felt that they were normal and I wasn't. Something normal people don't understand is that just being normal, average, unnoticeable, is the ultimate goal for anyone who stands out from the crowd for a reason they are ashamed of or embarrassed about. My skills in math and my positive experience playing basketball had given me more confidence, but would anything change back at the old school, or would I still be that stuttering, angry boy?

3

Special Class

Fourth grade was upon us. It was my first day back at Independence in over a year. The school looked exactly the same. I wondered if the students were, too. Our school went from kindergarten through fourth grade, so as a fourth-grader, I was one of the elder statesmen. In a sense, I was the big man on campus. By that time, I had grown another three or four inches and weighed as many as fifty pounds more than the next kid in my class.

I was surprised to find that my first day back to school was different from second grade. This time, I was sent to a separate part of the building to be in a "special class" with other special classmates. Many of my friends asked me where I was going, but I didn't know what to say so I didn't say anything. Instead I said, "I'll see you at lunch." I was too embarrassed and ashamed to tell them where I was really going. I thought to myself, "I must be stupid because I can't be in classes with my friends. Why do I have to stick out like a sore thumb? Why can't I be with my friends? That's where I want to be. I don't want to be with my special classmates. How am I going to keep avoiding my friends' questions?"

One day at lunch, Rick asked me how my new class was

going. I told him everything was going well even though I was thinking, "I hate being in these classes. I don't want you to think I'm stupid. I don't want to tell you the real reason I'm in these classes. I don't want you to know that I have a learning disability and it takes me longer to learn. I really just want you to like me so if I say everything is going well, then I know you will leave me alone and take me at my word." I didn't say anything for the rest of lunch; then Rick and I and a couple of kids from our table went out to play kickball on the playground. I remember feeling relieved that I had gotten through another situation without them finding out about my learning disability.

Later in the day, I saw Rick and some of my other friends again in gym class. Gym was the only class where I was mainstreamed, meaning I was included in the regular classes with the kids who used to be my classmates. They were happy to see me. I got a chance to laugh and hang out with them for a bit. Once gym class was over, I quietly walked away. Embarrassed and ashamed, I hoped no one would notice me going in the opposite direction of the fourth-grade class. But one of them did and yelled, "Hey, Bill! Where are you going?" At first, I didn't know what to say. Eventually, I just mumbled, "Uh, I have to get to my class." Fortunately, my friend just shrugged his shoulders and walked away. When I returned to my special class, I asked Mrs. Goodall why I couldn't be with my regular class. She didn't have an answer for me. All I knew was I had gym twice a week with the regular class from just two years ago. When I found out the reason I was in these classes was because I had a learning disability, I didn't understand what that meant. No one ever explained it to me. I just knew I was in special education classes and had to be there all day every day except for gym. How could I fix the problem when nobody would talk to me about it directly?

From time to time, my dad lost his patience with my stuttering. But I noticed whenever I was around him and didn't stutter, I would receive his approval and love. If I did stutter, however, I risked him yelling at me. I think he was nearly as frustrated as I was but didn't know how he could help. If I had known his feelings of frustration and helplessness, and he had known my frustrations and fears, maybe our relationship would have gone differently. Instead, my relationship with him consisted of a constant struggle to please him and avoid his anger. I also began to believe that other people weren't going to be patient enough to listen to me when I stuttered either, so when I talked to strangers, I tried to hurry up and say what I needed to say.

In addition to school, I played another year in the local recreational basketball league. I still hung out with my neighborhood friends after school. I wasn't getting into as many fights—probably because I wasn't around as many people in my special class. I still hated being in the special class separate from my regular class. I felt like an outsider looking in. I also still went to the playground at recess, but that year my friends never seemed to have recess when I did, so I was alone most of the time.

I got along with the kids in my special class, but I had no real interest in being friends with them. In my mind, they were the ones with real issues and the kids in the regular classes were the ones who thrived in their lives. My biggest problem was not wanting my friends or other classmates in the regular classes to think I was stupid or couldn't do the work. When I was with my special class outside of the classroom, I avoided making eye contact with anyone, especially those classmates I knew just a few years earlier. I worried they would make fun of me, think less of me or think I was stupid. I didn't know what my regular classmates thought of me, but I knew it had to be something bad.

I passed all of my classes in fourth grade. In fifth grade, I was again sent to a new school, and it was really hard on me. The nervousness I felt when I started at a new school made my stuttering uncontrollable. The school was called Sugar Grove and was made up of fifth and sixth-graders. Again, I was in special education classes. My class was on the first floor, right next to two doors leading out of the building. I still had some of the same classmates and some new ones as well.

My fifth-grade teacher was Mrs. Williston. She was a tall, thin, light-skinned African-American woman. The assistant teacher was Ms. Downington. Having a new school, new teachers, and some new students was not a good combination for me. I was discovering that I didn't do well in new environments. What I needed most was what any child at that age needs: consistency, routine, and friendship; but between changing schools and being separated from my friends, I got the opposite. Several of my new classmates made of fun of me, but the ones who knew me from elementary school stuck up for me. For that reason it didn't take long before all of my classmates in my special class stopped laughing at me.

I was still mainstreamed into gym class, but Mrs. Williston told me I had to behave and do my best or I would be taken out of it. Besides gym class, I was also in regular math classes in fifth grade. I still loved math because of the skills I acquired when playing with my baseball cards. I could do arithmetic in my head and show off my talents to my classmates and teacher. Again, my math ability took attention away from my stutter and put it on something that made them think, "Wow, I wish I could do that!" That was a nice change. I was now behaving in math and gym and doing fairly well in both. I noticed that the better I behaved, the more Mrs. Williston and Ms. Downington trusted and respected me.

I was doing well for several months and then I had a meltdown. One of my classmates in my special class stuck his tongue out at me and I lost my temper. This kid's name was Donny. He was an instigator. I wanted to beat him up. I walked over and pushed his seat backwards. He fell hard. Mrs. Williston rushed over and I was ready to fight her as well. I was uncontrollable by then, so some of my fellow class-mates came over and restrained me. I told them I was calm just so they would let me go long enough to kick Donny again. When Donny saw me coming, he ran to the back of the room and Ms. Downington got between us. Mrs. Williston called for one of the assistant principals to come down. By the time he arrived, I was calm and sitting behind a partition. That was our timeout area.

Mrs. Williston called my parents. My dad came to meet with my teachers. I received a three-day suspension. My dad yelled at me all the way home, using many words I was not familiar with yet. I spent those three days doing homework because I was grounded from playing with my neighborhood friends. I also had to apologize to Donny, my class, and my teachers when I returned to school.

I began to really hate school. I had nothing to look forward to there. Most of my time was spent in my special education classes. I wanted to be anywhere else. I looked around the room and wondered why I was there. I was smart. I just struggled in reading and writing and studying. I couldn't understand why I wasn't in more of the regular classes. I thought to myself, "Maybe it also has to do with my attitude. If I'm good in school, maybe Mrs. Williston will allow me to be in more of the regular classes with the people I know."

I always felt like my parents were punishing me by having me in those special education classes. It was now three years since I was in the same classes as the friends I had made in first and second grades. I rarely saw them, if ever. My life was a lot different from when I was younger, and I didn't like it. I just wanted to be back in the regular classes with the people I knew. I felt like an outcast. When I was at home, my parents seemed to yell at me more. I guess they were worried I was going to get kicked out of school for my bad temper and they would have to send me somewhere else.

My saving grace was being able to hang out with my

neighborhood friends, especially on the weekends. Between my friends and my brothers' friends, we had some great football games in our side yard. There were many weekends when these games would run two or three hours long. Then we would come back out and play at night, too.

At the time, I lived on a cul-de-sac with just three houses in a semi-circle. My house was to the left of the middle house. Our yard was about one acre. Although we played a lot of football in our side yard, we also played in our front yard, which neither of my parents liked much. My parents were concerned we might break a window, run into a lamppost, or run into the thin tree that was on the front side of the yard. There were definitely a lot of obstacles in the way, but that didn't stop us from playing football under the lights in our front yard. We called it Monday (or whatever night of the week we were playing) Night Football at Deering Stadium. If there was snow on the ground—or if it was still snowing—it just gave us another reason to play.

A typical football game inevitably involved my younger brother, Jamie, crying or leaving to go inside. I mean, who could blame him? He was only seven or eight years old at the time, and some of the kids he was playing with were six or seven years older than him. Jonathan, my older brother, told Jamie to suck it up, be tough, and play anyway. Sometimes that worked and other times it didn't. We also had our fights and temper tantrums. I was guilty of both, especially when I couldn't get my way. In spite of all that, we had a lot of fun playing football under the lights.

Our games usually began around seven in the evening and lasted until around eleven. Some of the best football we played was between my brothers and Peter and me. My friend Peter would do anything to win, even if it meant playing dirty. I liked that he was on my team. When the game took place during the day, sometimes a few friends would come in for lunch. When our games ended at night, we all went our separate ways.

One of the things I had in common with my brothers was that we were all big sports fans. My dad, my brothers, and I watched every Eagles game together, unless we went to my grandmother's house where we listened to them on the radio. Those were happy days for me, when I felt like a normal kid. Even my father would occasionally watch us with a smile on his face, and when I showed a little skill, I felt the acceptance that was so precious to me. But deep down, I knew it was because football didn't involve much talking.

4

Football at Deering Stadium

I had two grandmothers and one grandfather. My paternal grandfather died when I was a few months old. My mom's parents lived in South Jersey, which was about an hour from where we lived. At the time, all six of my first cousins also lived within an hour of us. My mom had two siblings—a sister and a brother. My mom's sister, who lived about twenty minutes from us in Flowerside, had four kids. Joel was the oldest, followed by Jake, Jarrod, and Paula. My mom's brother, Joel, and his wife, Lizzy, lived in South Jersey near her parents. They had two kids. Mary Joe was the oldest and Katie was a few years younger. I saw my cousins in Flowerside quite a bit since they were so close to me.

My dad also had two siblings. My Uncle Bob, and his wife, Aunt Marilyn, lived in a town about forty minutes away. They didn't have any children. My Aunt Rosie was a nun, so she obviously didn't have any kids. She was the principal of a Catholic elementary school. My dad's mom lived in Havertown, Pennsylvania, which was about forty-five minutes from where I lived. Grandmom Deering had my dad when she was forty years old. She was very active. She bowled until she was eighty-five. I saw both of my grandmothers quite a bit as an eleven-year-old kid.

I really looked forward to the holidays because I got to see all of my cousins. We usually met at Uncle Joel and Aunt Lizzy's house. That's where we had our Thanksgiving feast together. Since there were so many people at my uncle's house, not everyone got to sit at the "big table," which was code for the adult table. I sat at the kid table but I didn't mind. I usually made it a point to sit next to Mary Joe. She hated ketchup and I loved it. I loved grossing her out on Thanksgiving by putting ketchup on my turkey and mashed potatoes. I usually only used ketchup on hot dogs and fries, but I liked the reaction I got from her.

My Aunt Lizzy could bake like a champ. She made these BIG homemade chocolate chip cookies. I ate as many as I could until I was sick to my stomach and couldn't eat anymore. I always left her table full and satisfied.

While visiting with my cousins, grandparents, aunts, and uncles, I still had very little to say. No one in my family laughed at me, which was a big relief, but I still liked to keep to myself. My Uncle Joel always had the television turned to the pro football games that played on Thanksgiving. That's where I could be found. I wanted to watch the football games, drink soda, eat chips, and not talk, because every sentence was still a battle with my stutter. Typically, my cousin Jake and my brothers watched the games with me. The only time I really had to talk was when one of my aunts or uncles asked me a question, and then I did my best to answer with a yes or no. Other than that, I just smiled, watched television, ate a lot of food, and grossed out my cousins.

I got along well with all of my cousins, but I really liked speaking with two in particular. There was my cousin, Jake, who we all called Big Jake because he was so much taller than the rest of us. He was a basketball player. I felt very connected to him. He listened to me even when it would take me a few minutes to get out a word or two. I really appreciated when he listened because that kind of patience was rare in my life. Mary Joe and I got along well, too. She had a good sense of humor about me grossing her out and she was a great listener as well. She never interrupted me or became impatient with my stuttering, either.

Despite having no cousins on my dad's side of the family, I enjoyed visiting with my grandmother, Uncle Bob, Aunt Marilyn, and Aunt Rosie. Getting to my paternal grandmother's house was a pain in the neck because we had to take back roads and they were always jammed up with traffic. Grandmom Deering could really cook. She had a big sweet tooth, which my brothers and I appreciated. After dinner there were always plenty of choices for sweets, including ice cream, which was such a great treat for all of us. My brothers and I hardly ever had that kind of ice cream at home. We also had other options, such as chocolate chip cookies, cakes, and pies. My grandmother loved to bake. She would make us homemade chocolate chip cookies. They were always so good. Many times during our visits with Grandmom Deering, my dad, brothers, Uncle Bill, and I played cards. It was always a lot of fun and made me feel like a grown-up.

When I wasn't visiting my cousins, I saw Grandmother and Grandfather Baylor, which were my mom's parents. Grandmother Baylor could cook, too. She always made sure my brothers and I had enough food to eat, and she would give my mom any leftover sweets for us to take home. They lived approximately an hour from us. My brothers and I would often sleep in the car during the ride home. They were days full of peace and pleasure, but I have often wondered how much more I would have enjoyed them if I didn't need to hide my stutter with silence. I could have had long conversations with my grandparents, sharing my joys and fears, like my brothers and just about every other kid in the world were able to do.

5

Ride the Waves

Fifth grade was coming to an end and I was very happy the school year was almost over. I wondered when I was going to be out of special education classes. I didn't like them. The more I was around the other special kids, the less opportunity there was for me to hang out with the people in regular classes. I was still struggling in some academic areas like English and science, but I was getting tired of being in "special" classes. I thought they were supposed to be helping me improve in subjects that were difficult for me. At the end of fifth grade, our teachers, Mrs. Williston and Ms. Downington, told us they wouldn't be our teachers for sixth grade. I was disappointed because I had grown quite close to them. Despite being someone who acted out a lot, I liked the rigor and discipline they brought to their classes. They pushed me to do all of my homework. I didn't like that, but I knew it was important. My behavior was much better. I passed all of my classes.

Over the summer of 1979, my neighborhood friends, Chet and Bob, moved out of the area. Chet's family moved to Minneapolis. He was originally from North Carolina, so it wasn't the first time he had to move. I was sad to see them go. During that summer, my dad took my brothers and me deep-sea fishing. We went on a party boat down in Sea Isle City. That was a big treat for us. My dad had talked about taking us. It was exciting to finally do it! To get there, we had to leave early Saturday morning. At the time, Jamie was eight and Jonathan was fourteen. It took nearly two hours to reach the Jersey shore. My brothers and I had never been on a party boat before. It was a seventy-five-foot boat filled with kids and adults. We fished for the entire day. We brought sandwiches with us and bought sodas. It was a whole new kind of fun.

When we were on our way out to the deep waters, there was another adult sitting too close to my dad and he said something to us about it. He said, "Look at that shithead over there." My brothers and I all got a kick out of that because we were never sure what was going to come out of Dad's mouth. My dad didn't always have the best etiquette, but when he was blunt, he was funny. We still laugh about that today. When we arrived at our destination, we put our lines out and attempted to catch bluefish. They were very strong, even the small ones. The look on my brothers' faces as well as my own when we caught a fish was very satisfying for my dad. It was during times like these that I knew, even though we had our challenges, my dad loved my brothers and me.

My dad's mom had a ranch-style house with a quarter-acre of land near the boardwalk in Ocean City, New Jersey. Every summer she invited us to spend a week or two with her for our vacation. Her house had three bedrooms, one bathroom, and a sofa bed. Being in Ocean City also gave my brothers and I the chance to hang out with all of our cousins because they would come down, too. It was always a treat to go to the boardwalk and go on the rides. My favorite was the bumper cars. It was a fun way to take out my frustrations on my brothers and cousins. For once, we all had equal power and skill. My brothers enjoyed the scarier rides that went way up in the air, but I was afraid of heights. We all loved the beach, too. I wasn't a good swimmer, but I liked when I had the chance to rent a raft and ride the waves with my brothers. It was one of the few times my brothers and I didn't argue or fight. There was a lot of laughter. I didn't stutter when I laughed. I was normal. Happy.

Now, it was time to move on to sixth grade. I found there was a mix of old and new students in my special education class. There were fifteen students, which was the biggest class I had been in since my regular class in second grade. The lead teacher was Mrs. Crispi. She was very young—no more than twenty-five—and about five feet tall with curly black hair. Her assistant teacher was Mrs. Zachary. She was in her early sixties. She shared with us that she had been a teacher her entire life and that she really enjoyed it. Because of her age and experience, I found it odd she was the assistant to a twenty-five-year-old.

One of my classmates, Robbie, had a crush on Mrs. Crispi. At the end of each day, Robbie gave her a kiss on the cheek. Nowadays, that would be considered inappropriate behavior, but back in 1979, that kind of affection between teacher and student was acceptable. My other classmates and I got a kick out of Robbie's crush. Mrs. Crispi seemed to like it, too. I guess she saw it as someone caring about her and appreciating her for being a good teacher.

I continued to be mainstreamed in math and gym, but spent most of my day with my special education class. I still excelled in math class and behaved well in both math and gym. I still had a few meltdowns in my special education class, though. Luckily, there was a timeout room inside it—a cinderblock room that was so quiet I couldn't hear what was going on outside of it. I didn't have to go to the timeout room often, but when I did, I made sure to take advantage of it. Mrs. Crispi or Mrs. Zachary would come into the room every fifteen minutes to see if I was ready to come out and join the class again. Sometimes I would act mad to get more time in the room so I wouldn't have to be around my classmates or participate in class. They probably knew I was using the timeout room to get out of work, but they didn't care as long as I was better behaved when I came out.

I was still going to speech therapy, except now I wasn't going by myself. One of my classmates from math was in therapy with me as well. His name was Davidson. He was a twelve-year-old African-American boy and he stuttered, too, but not nearly as bad as I did. In fact, it was hardly noticeable. Being around Davidson turned out to be very good for me. Aside from discovering I wasn't the only person on Earth with this affliction, he was outgoing and fun. He encouraged me to keep going to speech therapy with him. I now had a reason to look forward to going—to hang out with Davidson.

I continued to play in the local basketball league. Our team wasn't that good. I think we won three or four games. But our win-loss record didn't really matter to me. I just enjoyed playing and being part of a team. Again, I knew no one would make fun of me for at least two hours and I could fit in and be a normal twelve-year-old. I also received an award at the end of the season as the most improved player in the league. My parents and I went to an award ceremony. My name appeared in the local newspaper. I was surprised to be recognized because I hadn't scored a lot of points. I suppose the people who decided to give me the award looked at other things like hustle, defense, and rebounds. I blocked a lot of shots because of my height, and I always hustled up and down the court. My dad attended all of my Saturday games from the time I started participating in second grade through eighth grade. It was a bit nerve-racking but I appreciated him being there and really wanted to impress him.

My grade school had an activity night every Friday throughout the school year. Anyone in fifth or sixth grade could go. It was a chance to hang out with some friends from my neighborhood and the people I knew from my math and gym classes. We played a lot of basketball. It was another opportunity for me to feel normal and not worry about someone making fun of me. There were girls that attended this event every week, but unlike my friends, I had no interest in meeting any of them. I was worried they would reject me outright when they heard me stuttering.

Mrs. Crispi and Mrs. Zachary made it very clear to our class from the beginning that neither of them would take any backtalk from the students. Mrs. Crispi had a system. She graded our performance every day based on how much we participated and how well we behaved in class. She created notes for each category. The best note to get was a "great" note, in which she would rave about our performance. The next best was a "good" note. The third was a "better" note. This is where Mrs. Crispi described improvements that were made, and areas that still needed work. My goal every day was to get a "great" note, but I didn't always achieve it.

In all honesty, sometimes I chose to act out just to get attention. On those days, I didn't listen or do any work. I did anything and everything to get myself in trouble. I broke my own records for time spent in the timeout room. Sometimes I sat in there for hours just to avoid being around others.

One time, I was so frustrated with Mrs. Crispi I asked if I could get a drink from the water fountain. After I drank as much water as I could, I left a mouthful of water in my mouth. When I returned to class, Mrs. Crispi asked if I had gotten enough water and I spit the water all over her face. I thought it was funny. My classmates thought it was funny, too. Mrs. Crispi didn't. A few of my classmates told me later that I had some nerve, which was like getting a pat on the back because they'd had their frustrations in the class, too. In the moment, what I did didn't seem like a big deal, but when Mrs. Crispi said, "Bill, I am going to call your dad and have him pick you up," I realized the impact of my actions.

When my dad arrived at Sugar Grove and Mrs. Crispi told him what I had done, he was furious with me. At the end of the conversation, I apologized to her. She accepted my apology, but my dad screamed at me all the way home. I was more scared of him than ever. He said, "Billy, wait until we get home." Sure enough, when we arrived at home, he whipped my butt. After that, I became a model student. I stopped getting into trouble and received a note every day that was either great, good, or better. I did all of my classwork and all of my homework.

My dad still had a hard time accepting my severe stutter and learning challenges. It didn't help that I was the opposite of my brothers, who excelled at everything. Jonathan, the oldest, was a ninth-grader at a private high school in the area. He was the starting running back for the football team and always got good grades. My parents trusted him enough to go to a Rolling Stones concert when he was just fifteen years old. He was a good kid and didn't have the challenges I had (although when he was very young, he needed surgery to remove a tumor). My younger brother, Jamie, was nine years old and in third grade at the time. He was a running back in the peewee league and scored several touchdowns. He also got good grades. I was the only one in my immediate or extended family who stuttered and had a learning disability.

I found out toward the end of sixth grade that many of my special education classmates were going to a new school district. I had gotten to know them since third grade. Some of them had done the work required to fully mainstream into regular classes for seventh grade. I was happy for them but sad for myself because I wasn't one of them. I dedicated myself to keeping up my good behavior so I might be fully mainstreamed as well.

The last week of school finally arrived and I was excited to be free for the summer. On the last day of school, Mrs. Crispi kissed every kid on the cheek on the way out, but just before my turn came, I ran by the other kids and out the door. I could see that she was disappointed, but I didn't care. As I walked down the hall alone, I wondered why I didn't care. She had been good to me. It wasn't until I was an adult that I understood why. I kept everyone at a distance without realizing it, because if someone I cared about ridiculed me, it hurt a lot more than if someone I didn't care about did it.

Over the summer, my Aunt Rosie and Grandmom Deering invited my brothers and I back to the Jersey Shore for five days. As usual, I couldn't wait to get on the bumper cars, and ride waves on inner tubes. Sometimes, when we were all exhausted after a day of play, my grandmother would splurge and buy us a pound of fudge or ice cream. My passion for fudge was matchless. We got vanilla, chocolate, and vanilla with nuts. It was amazing.

My parents didn't come with us this time. They told us before we left to be on our best behavior. They instilled in us at an early age that using curse words wasn't tolerated. They even considered "fart" and "hell" to be curse words. They ran a tight ship without exception.

We were with my grandmother and aunt one day and had been behaving when my brother upset me. Before I knew it, I yelled, "You are a f---ing a--hole." I was so angry that when my aunt told me not to talk like that, I also said something nasty to her. The minute it happened, she was on the phone with my dad. I spent the next few days like a prisoner on death row, knowing my punishment was waiting for me when I got home. Sure enough, within minutes of arriving home, my dad whipped my butt even more than he had after the water-spitting incident. One thing's for sure, I learned my lesson.

6

"B" is for Battleton

My first six years of grade school were behind me. It was time to move on to middle school. I was still in special education classes, but I had worked my way up to being almost fully mainstreamed. The last time that had happened was five years earlier when I was in second grade. Things were different now. For one, I was much taller. I had grown four inches over the summer. I was five feet, eleven inches tall as a seventh-grader. I was also at a new school, which meant I was going to stutter a lot more.

The school was unfamiliar and many of the kids were coming from different elementary schools. Even though I recognized several people from my class—and they recognized me—it had been five years since I had seen them and we had all matured a lot. To a certain extent, I was a stranger to them. All they knew was that I was now in their classes after a five-year gap. There was definitely an adjustment period. I had math, science, social studies, physical education, art, and lunch. My days were full. I still didn't say very much except in math class, the only class that gave me a chance to wow my classmates by adding or multiplying numbers in my head. Even my math teacher, Mr. Seers, was amazed by what I could do. I would probably like him now but at the time I found him a bit annoying. He had a saying he repeated over and over—so much so that I still remember it to this day: "CAN'T never did anything." I realized the truth of this simple statement when I was in eleventh grade.

In the fall, I tried out for the football team. Peter, my friend from the neighborhood, and a lot of people from my classes also tried out for the team. I made the team but rarely played. Our coach, Harry Magin, knew my brother, because Jonathan played for him a few years before me. Many of the eighth-graders on the team were big and strong, and so were many of the seventh-graders. Despite my size, though, I wasn't good at hitting, and enjoyed getting hit even less.

Every day after football practice, I had to take the bus home. I waited for the bus with other students who played sports. This simple activity became a nightmare because of my stuttering. My bus arrived and I got in and sat down. I was tired and anxious to get home when the bus driver announced, "To get off the bus, call out the name of your street and I'll stop."

I was afraid to talk and reveal my stuttering; I wondered how I would ever get off the bus. Because I had the most trouble with B's and D's, saying the name of my street, Battleton, was nearly impossible. The moment the bus driver said that, my chest became very tight, my heart started racing, and my breathing became shallow and rapid. I was so nervous I felt like I was going to poop my pants. I just wanted to get off the bus. I would rather have walked home in the pouring rain than face my fear of saying anything publicly. I knew if I spoke, I would immediately go from blending in with the other students to sticking out like a sore thumb.

The driver had to go to the high school to pick up the student athletes there as well. This gave me more time to delay the inevitable. Thoughts raced through my mind. "What am I going to do? It's not enough that I have to deal with my stutter all day. Now I have to figure out how I'm going to say the word Battleton? I wish I didn't stutter. Why can't I just talk normally like everyone else? Why does speaking have to be such a struggle for me? I don't know how I'm going to get off this bus. Let me take a look around to see if there is anyone who is getting off at my stop. Then he can say the name of the street."

As the bus pulled into the high school, however, I couldn't see anyone who would say the name of my street for me. The high school students got on the bus. Again, I looked around and there was nobody there who would be getting off at my stop. My mind continued to race. "What the hell am I going to do? How am I going to get off the bus? I can't say the name. I am going to stutter my head off. People are going to laugh at me. I don't want to be embarrassed. I don't want to be humiliated. I don't know what I'm going to do. I have to think of something."

As the bus driver pulled away from the high school, I decided to move from the middle of the bus to a seat at the front, right behind the bus driver. My plan was to repeat "Battleton" to myself over and over again. The bus driver made a left down Wagger Drive and then another left down Penny Way. By this time, students were calling out the names of their streets. "Whistler Lane," someone called. As we got closer and closer to my stop, I got more nervous. I wasn't sure my plan was going to work, but I was desperate. About twenty minutes into the bus ride, the driver made a left onto Morrison Road, which happened to be where my stop was located. Someone else called out, "Matter's Circle." The bus driver made the stop.

My stop was next. I must have repeated "Battleton" to myself at least two hundred and fifty times. We were about a hundred feet from my stop. I was so nervous sweat was pouring down my face, my heart was racing, my palms were sweaty, and I was literally shaking in my seat. When we were about twenty-five feet from my stop, I still didn't say anything. I was trying but I couldn't get the words out. Finally, I stood up and in a low voice so no one could hear me, said, "Um-um-um-um-um-um-um-um-um-um-um-um-um-um-um-um-um-um-b-b-b-b-b-b-b-b-a-a-a-a-a-a-a-a-t-t-t-t-t-t-t-l-l-l-l-l-ton. Um Battleton." I finally spit out the word right before the bus driver was going to pass my stop. The driver slammed on the breaks and opened the door. I gladly walked off the bus. The bus moved along and I crossed the street. I was so relieved to be off the bus. I thought there had to be an easier way to do this. I didn't want to go through that pain and anxiety for the rest of football season. I had to figure something else out.

The next morning, I got on my regular bus, but all I could think about on my ride to school was the terrifying experience from the day before. I was distracted at school all day because I knew I would have to take the after-school bus again. Now, I nervous about speaking in class, and I had the added anxiety of knowing I would have to look around my bus that afternoon, hoping to see someone who was getting off at my stop. All day I was thinking, "Maybe I'll skip football practice and just take the regular bus home. Maybe I'll walk home. It's only a thirty-minute walk at sunset. It won't be that bad. I'll stay on the sidewalk. I can definitely do that. Anything is easier than getting on that bus and struggling to get out the name of my street."

While I was at football practice, I was able to take my focus off stuttering and the after-school bus and just have fun with my teammates. I still had to deal with some of the eighth-graders on the football team laughing at my stutter, but I got through it. At the end of practice, though, reality rushed back in because I would have to take the bus. Again, I looked around for someone to save me, and this time found someone who was getting off at the stop before mine. But I was still very nervous so I asked this person if he would say the name of my street before getting off the bus. He said, "Bill, just get off at my stop and walk a little further." That's what I did. I got off at Matter's Circle, which was the stop before mine. It meant that I had to walk on Morrison Road, which was a busy street, for about a hundred yards, but I didn't mind. I was relieved because I didn't have to struggle to say the name of my street that day. I didn't have to practice saying the word "Battleton" in my head five hundred times. I didn't have to stutter or be embarrassed or humiliated. That day was a good day. On my walk home, I thought about how great it was to have someone make sure I was able to get off the bus. I was just happy to make it through another day, but I never knew what challenges the next day would bring.

There were good days, when someone would say the name

of my street or get off at my stop or the stop before mine, and there were bad days when I really struggled with stuttering and saying the name of my street was nearly impossible. There were days I would be so nervous about taking the after-school bus that I would be in the school bathroom sitting on the toilet every period of the day, paralyzed by fear. One of the effects of my fear was that I hardly ever ate breakfast because I was too anxious about the prospect of stuttering on the after-school bus, even though that would be ten hours later. I spent my days at school worried and distracted in every class except math, where I felt confident and was able to stand out in a good way for a change.

What started out as a hobby in second grade—creating math games with baseball cards by adding the statistics of various players in my head—ended up giving me a way to stand out and be popular with other kids. I continued to practice so my fellow classmates could forget about my stutter for a few minutes and see I had at least one thing going for me. I just wanted to be accepted by others so it helped to know that every day for at least one period I got to experience being liked, appreciated, and known. I really enjoyed when my classmates approached and said, "How did you do that? Can you teach me? I want to learn. You're amazing." When there was a multiplication or addition problem on the board, even my math teacher looked to me before solving it. Math was the highlight of my day. It was quite a contrast feeling like a fool on the bus and a boy genius in math class.

When math class was over, life abruptly returned to normal. The classmates who were so enamored with me went back to hanging out with their friends and I was once again alone and unknown—the student without a voice. People spoke to me only when they had to. I didn't attend any social events like school dances. I was so afraid of people laughing at my stutter, I felt like I was better off being invisible. Even though my teachers were patient with me, I often felt bad because it took me so long to get out my sentences and say what I needed to say. When speaking to them, I imagined what they might be thinking: "What am I going to do for Bill? He can't talk. How is he going to make it through this class? Does he ever not stutter? I wonder what the rest of his life is like. I feel bad for him. I wish there was more I could do for him. I wish he would talk more. He always seems embarrassed. I wonder if he is attending speech therapy. It must be really hard for Bill to go through school with such a severe stutter. I wonder how he copes with it." I didn't know what they were really thinking, though, because they never talked to me about it. It would have helped me if one adult was brave enough to break through my nervousness and try to support me. I don't know if they just didn't care enough, or if they thought ignoring my problem was what I wanted. I've heard that people who are grieving a major loss often complain that nobody mentions the name of the deceased to them. They act like it never happened. Maybe it's the same reason nobody mentioned my stuttering to me. We ignore each other's greatest pain, worried we'll make it worse.

English class was spent with my special education teacher. My writing and reading comprehension levels were low compared to my peers, so one period a day was spent with my fellow special education students. Besides math, English gradually became another class where no one laughed at me. Like many introverted kids, reading had become an escape for me, so I had pulled ahead of the crowd when it came to English and was respected and accepted by the other students in English class, too.

I often judged myself for being in special education classes because I thought it made me look stupid. To avoid embarrassment, I would sneak away or wait at my locker until my classmates went to their classes before heading off to my special ed classroom. I just wanted to be invisible. I now know most of them were probably too interested in their own lives and concerned with their own problems to obsess over mine. I was the one who constantly thought I was stupid because I stuttered. My whole life revolved around it. How could it not? No matter where I went, there it was, every time I opened my mouth. I couldn't get away from it even for a moment because communication with others is such a major part of everyday life, especially when we're in school. My stuttering was like a bully that found me no matter where I tried to hide.

My teachers interrupted me all the time when I stuttered, guessing what I was trying to say. They thought they were doing me a favor by interrupting and saving me from the struggle of stuttering, but they weren't. I would have preferred to stutter and spend the extra few minutes getting out my words so I could be heard instead of being interrupted over and over again. When they guessed wrong, I had to start all over again, which meant extra stuttering. I had thoughts like, "When are my teachers going to learn? Why can't they just wait for me to say what I want to say? Don't they know how frustrating and annoying that is for me? Why the hell do they keep doing that? Now I have to think about what I am going to say and practice it in my head over and over again, hoping that this time I won't stutter so badly that my teacher interrupts me again. Let me practice my breathing. Let me think of how I can say this without hitting on the sounds that give me the most difficulty."

The worst was when a student or teacher asked me my name. I'd start by saying, "My name is B-b-b-b-b-b-b-b-b-b-b-b-b-b-b-b-b-b-b-b-b-b-b-b-b...." and before I could get out the rest, the other students and my teachers would attempt to guess. "Bob? Brian? Bruce? Burt?" I'd say, "N-n-n-n-n-n-n-n-n-n-n-o-o-o-. No!" It was very frustrating for me. I couldn't understand why they couldn't just be patient and let me say my name. Nobody understood how challenging it was for me.

When someone asked me my name, my fear and thoughts

would start racing again. "I'm going to stutter. How can I get out of this? Can you just move on to the next person, please? What am I going to do? If I can just get beyond the first sound of my name without stuttering too badly then it won't be so horrible. I hope saying my name doesn't take me too long. I hope I don't repeat my sounds over and over again. If I get stuck on the *B* in my name, it's going to take me a long time to spit out the rest. I'll practice it to myself: Bill, Bill, Bill, I am Bill. My name is Bill. Okay, I have practiced my name over and over in my head a hundred times—let's give it another shot." But when I attempted to say my name as I had rehearsed mentally, it came out as, "My name is B-b-b-b-b-b-b-b-b-b-b-b-b-b-b-b-b-b-b-b-b-b-b-b-i-i-i-i-i-i-i-i-i-i-i-l-l-l-l-l-l-l-l-l-l. It is um-um-um-um-um-um-um-um-um-um-um-um-um-um-um-um B-b-b-b-b-b-b-b-b-b-b-b-b-b-b-b-i-i-i-i-i-i-l-l-l-l-l. My name is Bill." It literally took me two to three minutes to say my name. Stuttering continued to be the defining factor in my life, which brought with it embarrassment, humiliation, frustration, anger, sadness, isolation, low self-esteem, and the desire to be invisible.

I was almost six feet tall as a seventh-grader. I began to excel in gym class and feel equal to my peers. Mr. Lomas was my gym teacher that year. He was a recent graduate of Penn State University. He liked to joke around with everyone, including me. Even better, he always listened and never interrupted me. After so many impatient teachers, or teachers who mistakenly thought it helped me to guess what I was trying to say, I really appreciated that. By this time, being interrupted had become one of my biggest concerns when speaking with teachers and people I didn't know. My special education teacher and speech therapist were two other people I could count on to be patient and let me say what I wanted to say. They had a lot of compassion for me. In fact, more than I had for myself.

I started to "rate" my stuttering. Any time I spoke in my classes, which wasn't very often, I would spend the rest of

class consumed with thoughts like, "I wonder what my classmates thought of my stutter today? Was it better or worse? I
think I spoke better, not too many um's. I didn't block on too
many words. I didn't repeat my sounds over and over again.
This time it was only five times, not fifty. I wish I didn't stutter.
I wish I didn't get embarrassed. I wish the teacher wouldn't
call on me. I wish I could just speak normally like everyone
else. Then my life would be easier and people would like me."
I imagined what my classmates must be thinking: "Why can't
he say the words like everyone else? Doesn't he know how
easy it is to speak? He must be stupid. Man, why does it take
him so long to get out his words? Sometimes he's pretty good
and other times he can't say one freaking syllable."

If I didn't stutter at all when answering a question, it was
a miracle. I had such a high when that happened. On those
rare occasions, I would sit confidently in my chair with my
chest out, thinking to myself, "YEAH!!!!!!!!!!!!!!!!!!!!!!!!!!!!! I
didn't stutter! Life is good. I am so proud of myself. I want a lot
more of these moments!" But those moments were short-lived
because it was never long before another moment of extreme
stuttering would occur. When I say extreme, I mean having to
sound out each word. Sometimes I even had to spell the word
out or write the word down on a piece of paper. Those were
the moments I dreaded the most. Most of my classmates sup-
pressed laughter. Others made no effort to hide it and laughed
out loud. I wanted to run out of the room and keep running
until I found someplace where I could live my life alone, never
having to speak to anyone ever again. My teachers didn't know
what to do other then tell my classmates to stop laughing at me.
I remember wishing there was a place I could go where I could
learn how to talk and come back when my stutter was gone.

None of my classmates stuttered that year. They had no
concept of my daily struggle from one moment to the next;
from one class to the next; from walking to my bus stop in
the morning to taking the after-school bus in the evening. As

far as I knew, my classmates had never even met anyone who stuttered. Fortunately, the classmates I had known since grade school didn't laugh at me; only certain kids did—usually the students who came from other elementary schools and who didn't know me. I would often wonder why they laughed and why they couldn't just accept me as I was. I was just like them except for my stutter. I still wanted to beat up the classmates who laughed at me because I wanted to make them feel how much they had hurt me. Anytime they laughed at me or smirked or said, "Did you hear him? He c-c-c-c-c-c-a-n't t-t-t-t-talk," I wanted to slam their faces against the lockers. I thought that would make them leave me alone. In the end, to avoid getting in trouble for fighting again, I kept my mouth shut and stayed angry and frustrated in silence. I had more self-control, but I still bullied myself. Nobody ever thought as little of me as I thought of myself.

7

Playing the Game

Sports continued to be the great equalizer for me, where I could stand out because of my hustle and have fun hanging out with friends on my street. Everyone accepted me. People knew me as more than the kid with the severe stutter. Being a part of the basketball league really helped me to be less isolated, too. I wasn't as aggressive as some of the other kids in the league, but I really didn't care about how many points I scored. I played to be with non-judgmental friends and take the focus off my stuttering. My coach and teammates were all very understanding. I tried out for my school basketball team but was cut, which was very disappointing for me. My disappointment didn't last long, though, because I knew I could still play in the recreational league. My coach was Mr. Lewis. He was originally from Kentucky. He had a bit of a southern drawl. His son, Burt, was on the team. He was my age.

Mr. Lewis was the first coach who was hard on me and really pushed me. He taught me how to box out for a rebound and play defense. He wanted me to play hard and be aggressive. I really didn't like playing that way, but he kept pushing me to do it, so I listened. I was blocking a lot more shots. I was moving more and playing defense. I was still hustling up and down the court but now I was scoring points and rebounding, too. Our team was good. We won nine out of ten games during the regular season and ended up winning the league championship. I also made the thirteen-year-old traveling all-star team, which was very exciting because I had never made an all-star team before. Burt made it, too. He was a guard and played very well. He was the leader of the team, which I can imagine made his dad proud. In the end, I was glad Mr. Lewis pushed me. He was one of the coaches for the all-star team, too. I didn't play much but I didn't care. It was thrilling just to be on the team. I did get into one game and scored two points. That was thrilling, too, and no one ever made fun of me.

I spent a lot of time by myself when I was at home because my dad was still hard on me. I stayed in my bedroom after uncomfortable interactions with him, or just to avoid him entirely. When he yelled at me because of my stutter, I got angry and wanted to curse him out, but I never did. I would lay in my bed, thinking, "My dad has no idea what it's like to stutter. He doesn't know about the struggles I go through. He doesn't know how difficult saying one word or one sentence is for me. He doesn't know how often I have to repeat a sound or a word in my head before I try to say it. If he did, he would shut his mouth and show me some compassion. He has no idea how much pain I go through in my day-to-day life."

I was not able to express any of these thoughts to my dad. I imagined he would say, "Billy, you're making that up. That's not true. It isn't really that hard for you." Sometimes I wondered how he would react if he was forced to deal with my severe stutter for a day. If our roles were reversed, how would he feel if I told him to "spit out the f---ing words"? I wanted to beat him up when he yelled at me for stuttering. No matter what I did, I never felt I could do enough to make him proud of me.

My mom was the peacemaker. Something I couldn't understand at the time was that I stuttered badly with my dad but didn't stutter at all with my mom. No matter how badly I stuttered throughout the day, I could come home and speak with my mom and never stutter. It was the weirdest thing. She was the only person I never stuttered around. That isn't to say I had long conversations with her. I didn't talk much. I was still happy saying as little as possible. The only reason I left the house was to play sports in my neighborhood, when I could forget about my stutter and just focus on the game.

8

Inspired

If the fear of stuttering hadn't stopped me as a seventh-grader, I would have spent a lot less time in my bedroom and more time socializing with friends in my neighborhood. I would have introduced myself more often instead of shying away from people who I thought might laugh at my stutter. Maybe I would have even made a run for class president. Instead of living in fear, I would have been living my life with courage.

Middle school would've been quite different for me if had I been introduced to a speaker who stuttered and shared his pain, struggles, and triumphs. Hearing from someone else who went through the same struggles as me would have helped me realize that I didn't have to be so hard on myself. I would have realized that I didn't have to judge myself for stuttering or feel embarrassed or ashamed about it. I wouldn't have felt like I had to be quiet and accept all the teasing. I would have had the courage to stop getting angry, stop expressing myself with my fists, and ask my classmates to stop laughing at me and show me some compassion. I would have realized that I didn't have to let my fear of stuttering stop me in life. I would have taken more risks, such as raising my hand and answering questions in class or going to school dances.

If my fellow classmates had heard an adult with a stutter, who went through the struggles I went through, they may have been much more compassionate and understanding toward me. It would have been interesting to find out what my classmates learned from a speaker who stuttered. Maybe they would have opened up to me about their own struggles, insecurities and challenges. It would have been very interesting to learn about their struggles. Even though they didn't stutter, I bet they had their own version of "stuttering" in their lives.

A Diversity Day would have been even better. It would have been similar to Career Day, except instead of careers options, there would have been booths for different types of disabilities, different nationalities and different gender orientations. Students would have had the opportunity to learn about the daily struggles of the school friends they thought they knew. Students, teachers, and administrators would have had the chance to ask questions and learn something from the answers.

If I had heard from an adult who had struggled academically because of a learning disability and the steps he had taken to overcome his challenges would have helped me see ways to overcome my learning disability. Hearing from an individual who dealt with being bullied may have instilled in me more concern about others rather than being so focused on myself. Maybe someone who did the bullying could speak as well so others could understand and identify the problems that give rise to that behavior, too. In most cases, bullies are lashing out because of personal problems or traumas, as I was.

Instead of just one day, imagine if every middle school student learned about diversity during a one-year class. Speakers would come in to share their experiences based on that week's topic. Rather than being graded on exams, students would write a paper each week on what they had learned from the speakers and what new actions they were going to take so they could support others who were different from them.

At the end of the year, there would be a one-week celebration of diversity. The students would choose five speakers who had made the biggest impact on them, and each speaker would come back for one of the five days that week to emcee the program.

The highlight of this program would be the students. They would express themselves through artwork, music, spoken word, and public speaking regarding how the program had made an impact on them. Students would express what they had learned about themselves and others, what new goals they had created for their lives, and how they would support others.

Exposure to a variety of speakers would have really made a difference for me. I could have been there for my friends and listened to them, too. I couldn't even tell you what their struggles were because I was so focused on mine. My struggles were obvious every time I attempted to speak. I would have discovered that I wasn't the only one who was struggling. I imagine there were many others silently enduring challenges that weren't as visible as mine.

My classmates on the bus may have opened up and shared their daily challenges with me. If I had started building relationships with the people on the bus, I would have felt confident that I could get off the bus at my stop because they would have had my back. I would have had more friends who listened to me and stood up for me if necessary. That would have been a much different experience, and not just for me but for them as well.

I believe a diversity program like that would result in much less bullying. Acceptance and tolerance would rule the day. Students would be free to be themselves and they would learn to have empathy, compassion, generosity, and love for themselves and others. A school with this program would be known for all the right reasons. Students, teachers, administration, and the community would all thrive. The traditional academic subjects are all important but without compassion, school can become a place of trauma, anxiety, and bullying.

9

Not Quite Out of the Woods

I stuttered severely from first through seventh grades, so when I started eighth grade, I noticed a difference right away. My stutter almost completely vanished. I couldn't explain it. I think I finally felt safe, like I didn't have anything to worry about. It felt so good to speak normally. I wasn't hesitant to raise my hand in any of my classes. That's not to say I started raising my hand, but the fear of raising it and getting called on wasn't there anymore. It was a monumental relief after all those years of anxiety. I felt comfortable in all of my classes and I felt confident. I still played on the football and basketball teams. Since I wasn't stuttering, I didn't have to worry about taking the bus home like I did as a seventh-grader. My home life was better, too. My dad wasn't yelling at me to spit out my words. I hung out with friends in my neighborhood more. Overall, my life was going well. Long-term friendships, stability, caring teachers, coaches and speech therapists, repeated success in sports and academics, and the ongoing support of my mother all contributed to me finally being able to speak without stuttering.

I wasn't out of the woods yet—far from it—but I had made

great strides from I was that second grader whose frustration and confusion compelled him to beat up others.

In the fall of 1982, I began my high school career at Wissahickon. Since my stutter went away completely in eighth grade, I was feeling confident and optimistic. I felt that if I didn't stutter, I didn't have anything to worry about. Then I had my first few days of school and discovered that all of my self-confidence was gone. My stutter was back in a profound way. I couldn't say anything without terrible difficulty. People asked me my name and it would take me minutes to get it out. In that amount of time, I would attempt to say, "Bill" a minimum of one hundred times, and "um" several times as well, before finally being able to say my name. All of my childhood embarrassment came roaring back. The bully had found me again just when I thought I was finally free of him. The laughing, whispering, and pointing started again, too. I didn't like that kind of attention. My face turned bright red, sweat poured down it, and I just wanted to disappear again. I was devastated.

After mysteriously losing my stutter in eighth grade and getting it back again in ninth, I felt as if I had been released from prison, tasted freedom, then thrown back into my old cell. Every single day, I went to school worried about whether people were going to laugh at my stutter, anxious that if the teacher called on me in class I wouldn't be able to get the words out. I was petrified that I would be embarrassed, humiliated, and drenched in sweat like that eight-year-old kid I had been years ago. I couldn't believe I was back to being nervous about classmates asking me my name because I knew I wouldn't be able to say it. What's worse than not being able to say your first name? So, to keep that from happening, I avoided direct eye contact with as many people as possible.

After a few weeks of ninth grade, I fantasized about returning to the glory days of eighth grade when I had magically lost my stutter. I wanted to hide once more so I wouldn't have to talk to anyone. It didn't take long for all of my anxiety, worry, and frustration to return. I felt like an eight-year-old all over again. I stopped eating breakfast again because I was so nervous about going to school and having someone make fun of me.

I had one class with upperclassmen. When I had to introduce myself, they laughed and called me stupid under their breath. I thought they would be more mature and set an example of respect and compassion. I was wrong. I wished my stutter would go away like it had before. I wished people would show me compassion. I wondered why they couldn't understand I was doing my best to get my words out.

Again, I only felt free and confident in math class. I had continued to practice and had developed my calculation skills even more. I could now add, multiply, subtract, and divide numbers in my head quicker than the teacher could arrive at a solution using a calculator. For one period a day, I didn't have to wish for invisibility. I didn't have to fade into the background without anything to offer. I got to shine. For one period a day, I got to be accepted by peers who were amazed by my abilities. I was able to be a real and even extraordinary person, not just "that guy who stutters." I didn't have to worry about my stutter there, either. My peers were patient with me, probably because they respected me for something else. When math class ended, just as before, I turned back into the person with a severe stutter; the person no one respected.

Not much had changed at home, either. I still had to deal with my dad yelling at me. He was going through a difficult time in his life. He didn't have a job and started drinking a lot. He seemed to take his anger out on me. I was the one who got yelled at the most.

10

Oral Presentation

All I ever seemed to hear about during my freshman year was a history teacher named Mr. Lazarus. "You've got to get Mr. Lazarus. He is so cool. He's friendly and he takes students on field trips to the Italian market." Well, in my second semester, I got the esteemed Mr. Samuel Lazarus for history. He seemed like a nice guy. He joked around with everyone and all the students seemed to like him. Then, in one of my first classes, he stated, "Everyone will have to do a three-minute oral presentation in a few months." I was stunned. I nearly fell out of my chair. I immediately became a nervous wreck and struggled to come up with a way to get out of it. I resolved that I would simply explain to Mr. Lazarus that I can't do an oral presentation because I stutter. Surely he would understand my reasoning, I thought. Surely he wouldn't want me to stutter on every word and be embarrassed.

Whenever I was assigned an oral presentation in previous grades, I just told my teachers I stuttered and got to write papers instead. Doing a written assignment was such a relief. My teachers had always given me a pass. I didn't listen to anything else Mr. Lazarus had to say that day. I was too overcome by fear of having to potentially stutter in front of a whole new group of people.

At the end of the class, I approached Mr. Lazarus and said, "My-my-my-my-my-my-my-my-my-my-my-my n-n-n-n-n-n-n-n-n-n-a-a-a-a-a-a-a-a-a-a-a-m-m-m-m-m-m-m-m-m-m-m-e is b-b-b-b-b-b-b-b-b-b-b-b-b-b-b-i-i-i-i-i-i-i-i-i-i-i-i-i-i-i-i-i-i-i-l-l-l-l-l-l-l-l-l-l-l-Bill D-d-d-d-d-d-d-d-d-e-e-e-e-e-e-e-e-e-e-e-e-e-r-r-r-r-r-r-r-r-i-i-i-i-i-i-i-n-n-n-n-n-n-g-g-g-g-g Deering. If you haven't n-n-n-n-n-n-n-n-n-n-n-n-n-n-n-oticed, noticed, I st-st-st-st-st-st-st-st-st-st-st-st-st-st-utt-utt-utt-utt-utt-utt-er, stutter. Is there any w-w-w-w-w-w-w-w-w-w-w-w-w-w-w-w-w-w-w-way I could do a wr-wr-wr-wr-wr-wr-wr-wr-wr-wr-wr-wr-wr-itten paper?"

Mr. Lazarus turned to me and said, "No, Bill. I think it would be a really great idea for you to do an oral presentation." He then returned to his work, clearly indicating that the conversation was closed. I stood there stunned with disbelief for a few moments before walking away with my head down, devastated. I was trapped. It was like finding out I was going to be executed by a firing squad. That may sound like an exaggeration, but as a young person, acceptance is everything. The thought of presenting in front of my entire class of thirty students was terrifying. I went home and cried in my room.

My mom came in a few minutes later and asked, "Bill, what's wrong?"

"My history teacher told me I have to do a three-minute oral presentation in a few months."

"Bill, didn't you explain to your teacher that you stutter?" she asked.

"Yes, I did, Mom," I answered, "and he said he thought it would be a good idea."

My mom said, "Bill, just practice in the mirror. That will help." Her words were comforting to me, but it didn't take away my fears about having to present to a group of thirty students. The only comfort I felt was knowing I still had a few months to prepare.

I struggled to think of ways to get out of the oral exam—flu, pneumonia, malaria—but finally had to deal with the reality of doing it, mainly because everyone who knew I was terrified by it, especially Mr. Lazarus, would know I was lying. I decided to take my mom's advice and practice in the mirror. It sounded good in theory. Every night I prayed to God to take away my stuttering. I asked God to give me anything else besides stuttering; but nothing changed.

Wherever I went, stuttering was always there. Everyone takes for granted saying "hi" and "hello" and "how's it going" to each other, but even that was a struggle for me. And it wasn't just me not saying hello to anyone; students who knew about my stuttering didn't say hello to me—probably because they knew it would embarrass me to try and answer. The result was a silent world. I watched others and wondered how it felt to simply sit and have a casual, light-hearted conversation, envying something that most people on earth enjoy naturally—being able to just say what's on their minds. My only relief came when I was by myself or with my neighborhood friends. I could stutter as much as I wanted with them. They accepted me.

I spent a lot of time thinking about what it would be like not to stutter. I would have been friends with everyone in my high school. I wouldn't have had to hide all the time. I wouldn't have had to ask my teachers not to call on me. I would have had the self-confidence to make new friends. I would have been able to play sports in school, not just the public recreation league. I would have been liked.

My parents argued with each other about my stuttering a lot. My mother didn't like it when my dad came down hard on me. She remembered her own childhood stuttering so well, she knew it was useless for him to tell me, "Billy, just spit the words out. Think about what you're going to say and say the

51

words!" That was easy for *him* to say. He couldn't understand why I couldn't speak normally, but he didn't have the will to study and understand it, either.

My French teacher didn't care that I stuttered and called on me several times throughout the semester. The problem was I never knew *when* he was going to call on me. It was always a surprise. I was constantly on the edge of my seat, worried he was going to say my name and I would have to answer a question. When he did call on me, I usually stuttered severely and my classmates laughed, as usual. I couldn't wait for that class to be over. It was the only class in which I had to speak to earn participation credit. In my other classes, the teachers just let me listen and only called on me when I absolutely had to say something. I appreciated that. Still, it seemed like many people thought stuttering was somehow optional; that I was doing it for attention, or that I could just conquer it with sheer willpower.

One of the most difficult aspects of my classes was when my teachers took roll call and I had to say, "here." Again, the simplest things for everyone else were very challenging for me. As my teachers did roll call, I practiced saying the word "here" over and over again in my head before it was my turn to speak. Even then I usually didn't say, "here." I said, "Um, here." Then came the looks and comments from my class-mates. Sometimes I would overhear them.

"Did you hear him? He said 'um, here.' How hard is it to say here?"

Then anger would rise in me and, again, I would think, "They have no idea what I go through just to say one word. You would think they would be able to show me some com-passion. Is that too much to ask?"

Lunch was one period of the day where I didn't have to talk to anyone. I always brought my lunch. There was no way I was going to buy my lunch because that would mean having to stutter and deal with embarrassment. Anything to avoid that. Sometimes I sat with people I knew would leave me alone. Other times I would eat by myself. The times I ate by myself were hardest. Even though I didn't have to worry about people laughing at me, I was more worried about having my classmates think I didn't have any friends; that I was all alone. I spent a lot of my time worrying about what other students thought of me and wondering if they would ever be able to look beyond my stutter. When lunch was over, it was off to history class with Mr. Lazarus.

After a few weeks of Mr. Lazarus announcing that everyone would be doing an oral presentation, I finally came to terms with the fact that I would have to face my fears and do one of my own. It was still several weeks away, and I had to get my research done on the person I was going to discuss. Each of us had to pick a person; I got Voltaire. After several weeks of researching and taking notes, I had an outline for my presentation. Once I had that, I began practicing in the mirror like my mom had suggested. It felt weird, but after a few times, I got used to it. Even though I was by myself, I still stuttered severely. I thought, "If I am stuttering this badly by myself, how am I going to be able to get up in front of a group of thirty students and do it?" But I kept practicing over and over again in the mirror until I had my presentation down and felt confident that I could deliver it without stuttering.

After several weeks of practicing, I didn't stutter at all the last few times. I really didn't care about the material I was going to present or about the grade I would receive. I just cared about getting through my presentation without stuttering. The only thing that mattered was finding a way to avoid being laughed at.

Words cannot really convey how nervous I was about presenting in my history class on the day of my talk. I wasn't able to eat anything at all, and I had to use the bathroom every period that day because of my nervous stomach. In addition, my mind wandered during all of the classes leading up to my presentation. I mean, who could blame me? It was the first time in my fifteen years of existence that I was going to have to do an oral presentation, and I hoped it would be the last.

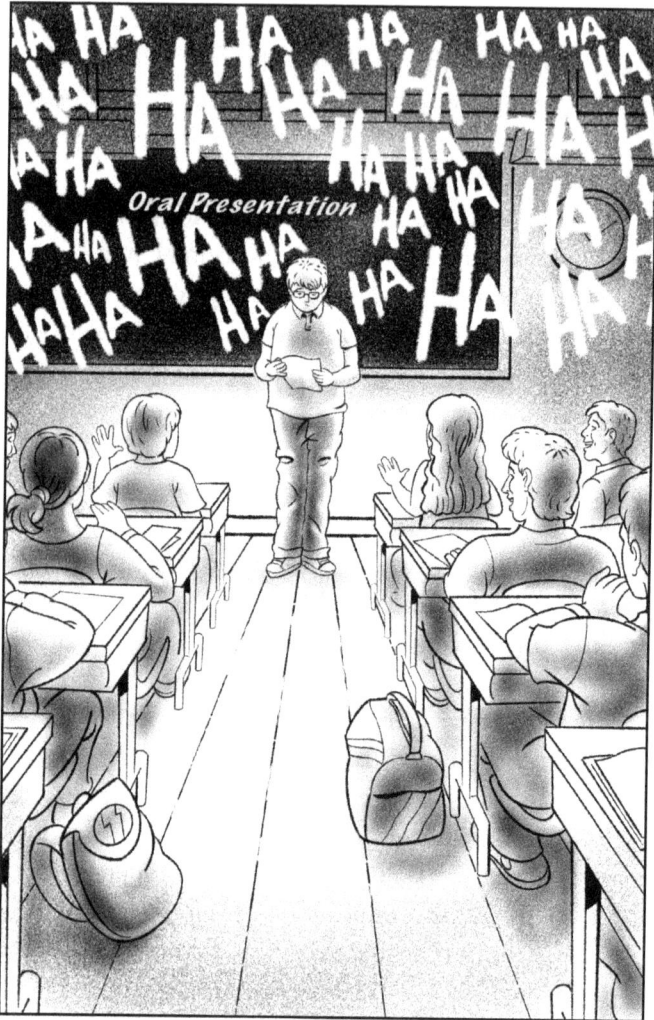

As usual, there wasn't anyone else in my class or the school who stuttered. I figured my classmates were nervous about doing their talks, but their concerns were different. They didn't have to worry about whether they were going to stutter on every syllable of every word. In all my classes, my teachers would say things like "make the best of it" or "slow down and take your time." My favorite one was, "Deering, relax!" This always made me think, "Relax? Wow! Why hadn't I thought of that? All these years of stuttering and that's all I need to do? Okay, I'll start right now!" I knew they were trying to help, but none of those comments did. Their comments just made me more nervous. I didn't blame my teachers, though. They had my best interest in mind, but it was very frustrating.

I finally got to history class on oral exam day. As I slowly walked to Mr. Lazarus' class, every step was filled with dread. I expected someone to yell, "Dead man walking!" It was my last class of the day. He was very friendly and greeted all of his students outside the door. When we were all seated, he said, "Today is the day we begin our oral presentations." I looked around at the thirty other people in my class and thought to myself, "There is no way all of us are going to be able to go today." That was comforting because there was a good chance I might not get called on.

Mr. Lazarus began the presentations by asking, "Is there anyone who wants to volunteer to go first?" Of course, there were a few students who were either excited to do their talk or just wanted to get it over with. Those students went first. After that, Mr. Lazarus randomly picked people to go, which meant I had no idea when or if I was going to be picked. His method was nerve-racking.

I looked up at the clock and noticed there were only about twenty-five minutes left of class. My chances of not being called on that day seemed good. Then Mr. Lazarus said, "Bill Deering, it is your turn to go." At first, I was stunned. I couldn't believe I actually had to do this talk. I stood up out of my chair and walked to the front of the room. Even after all I had already been through, the feeling I had during that short walk was very unfamiliar to me. It seemed like a long walk even though it was only about twenty feet. When I got to the front of the room, I turned around and looked at all of my classmates. Sweat was pouring down my face. My heart was racing and my knees were literally shaking. Then, Mr. Lazarus said, "Are you ready to go?" And I nodded.

In that moment, I thought, "How am I going to pull this one off without stuttering?" All thirty of my classmates stared at me silently. I opened my mouth and attempted to speak. I say attempted because it took me almost a full minute to get out my first word. Whatever confidence I had was gone. I thought to myself, "Here we go again." It was not a good start. I had no idea what to do. I knew I was going to stutter badly the entire time. I resolved myself to just muddle through it so I could sit down again.

About three or four minutes into my presentation, I noticed that my classmates started laughing. That made my stutter worse. The harder I attempted to get the words out, the worse my stutter became. I fought through it and delivered my talk the best that I could. There were full sentences in which I didn't stutter at all and then there were words and sentences that took me up to a minute to get out of my mouth. My presentation was supposed to be three minutes, but that was for someone who didn't stutter. It took me twenty minutes.

My classmates laughed at me through the entire talk. Mixed in with their laughter, I heard the words stupid, retarded, and idiot. I don't think Mr. Lazarus heard them because he wouldn't have stood for that kind of disrespect, but I heard them loud and clear. By the time I finished, my shirt was soaked with sweat. All I wanted to do was run out of the room and never return. I decided in that moment that I was never going to speak again. I was devastated. It was the worst experience of my life. Again, I wondered how people could laugh at someone with an obvious handicap and still consider themselves good people. I wondered why they couldn't be more mature than that. And I wished they could show me just a little compassion.

After that class, the school day was over, which meant I got to go home. I got on the bus, got off at my stop, and walked home. When I walked into the house, my mom asked me how my talk had gone. At first, I didn't want to tell her. It was too embarrassing. Then I broke down and said, "It was the worst day of my life. I stuttered so badly, Mom. My presentation took me twenty minutes instead of three and all the students laughed at me."

My mom said, "Bill, I am sorry that happened, but you did get through it and I am proud of you for that."

I told her I wasn't going to talk at school anymore.

"Why not?" she asked.

"I don't want to go through the pain of people laughing at my stutter. I would rather be quiet than run the risk of having people make fun of me."

My mom didn't know what to say. I went to my bedroom and struggled to process what had happened. I thought, "Why couldn't I be fluent? I practiced and practiced over and over again in the mirror. I felt confident going into my talk. But practicing alone is different than doing it in front of a group. Why did I think I could actually deliver a talk without stuttering? I must have been crazy. I stutter very severely and that is how it's always going to be for me. I might as well get used to it. I might as well accept that regardless of how hard I try, people will always laugh at me. I am done speaking in class. I am never going to open my mouth in school again."

The next day in school, I kept the promise I had made to myself. I didn't speak in any of my classes. In fact, I went to my teachers and asked them not to call on me unless I absolutely had to answer a question. Most of them honored my request. My French teacher and Mr. Lazarus were the two that did not. I dealt with it as best as I could.

A few days after my talk, my older brother, Jonathan, asked me how my presentation had gone and I told him what happened. He said, "Bill, I'm sorry to hear that." Then he said something that surprised me. He said, "Bill, stuttering is not a big deal. People don't care about your stutter."

At the time, that comment really hurt. I knew he meant well, but I couldn't help thinking, "He has no idea what he's talking about. What does he mean stuttering is no big deal? How would he know? He's just like my father. He doesn't understand the kind of pain and frustration I go through every day. He has no idea how embarrassing it is to stutter on every syllable of every word. For him to say that, he must be clueless to the feeling of all those eyes looking at me while I struggle to get out my first name. Maybe for him stuttering is no big deal, but for me stuttering is very real and the most frustrating part of my life."

I was really pissed off at my brother, but I didn't tell him how I felt. In fact, that was how I lived my life in ninth grade. Rather than standing up for myself about stuttering, I decided to say nothing. By saying nothing, I let my classmates believe it was fine for them to mock and bully me. But inside, I was very angry. I often thought about what it would be like to stand up to my classmates and tell them off, but knew I would stutter doing that too. I considered reverting to my grade school tactics and pushing them into lockers or just telling them to shut up. They had no idea what I went through just to speak. They had no idea that I practiced my answers over and over again just in case I got called on, or how my only hope was that practicing would help me be fluent, even though that very rarely happened.

I didn't even consider going to the principal or the vice-principal with my issue. What could they do? It was my word against someone else who could actually speak and, in many cases, an upperclassman. In my brief experience in high school, upperclassmen had the respect of the administration while freshmen were just trying to get through. It was another layer added to my feeling that I didn't have a voice.

My daily routine after the disastrous presentation was

about the same. I continued to say very little to anyone. I was still extremely nervous, anxious, and worried, except now I didn't have the occasional outlet of talking even with friends. I avoided making eye contact. When a teacher looked my way, I put my head down or looked away. I didn't want to have anything to do with anybody. I thought, "What's the point? Everyone laughs when I speak anyway." I just wanted to get through the day without being ridiculed. When that happened, I considered it a great day. If by chance one of my teachers called on me and I said the answer fluently, that was a major victory for me too. When I didn't stutter, I was on top of the world, unstoppable. Unfortunately, that rarely happened. Most days, when I had to speak for some reason, I was mocked, bullied and intimidated.

Even though I was quiet, other students knew I stuttered and found ways to let me know about it. I could rarely walk down the hall without someone doing an impression of me stuttering. Again, I never said anything. I wanted to but a lot of the bullies were bigger than me and I let that stop me from standing up for myself. As a result, I would go home angry, frustrated, resentful, tired, sad, but most of all, lonely. I was happy when the weekends came because that gave me a break from the taunting.

I still avoided social events and dances. I feared being laughed at by girls even more than guys. Asking a girl to a dance is nerve-racking for most guys, but for me, just being at a social event and trying to talk was a monumental challenge. I never asked a girl to a dance or anywhere else. I was paralyzed by my stutter and unwilling to step beyond my fears. My thinking was: "I would rather be safe at home by myself than risk people making fun of me at social events."

11

Food Becomes My Friend

Weekends still gave me a chance to hang out with my neighborhood friends and play sports like football or basketball. While that part of my weekends was great, being at home was becoming increasingly difficult. The yelling matches between my parents had become more frequent. They were mostly about the fact that my dad didn't have a job and wasn't looking for one. He spent his days watching television, which really pissed my mom off. She got a job and supported him as well as us. I knew my dad drank now and then but I didn't know the full extent of it.

I became increasingly angry with my dad. Eventually, I started to avoid him. Around that time, my dad started sleeping in the extra bedroom. I dreaded going home after school because I knew I would have to see him. I prayed he would be in a good mood so he would be patient with me because he always asked me about my day. I answered him only when I had to. Sometimes he would yell so I would say "good" or "okay." I kept it as short as I could. I think he just didn't know how he could make a difference for me. Since his two other sons didn't stutter and did well in school, I was a mystery to him.

My older brother, Jonathan, was now a senior at a private

high school in Philadelphia. He still thrived on the football field as the starting running back. He also excelled on the baseball field. He was offered scholarships for both sports. He was the first-born child. It seemed like he could do no wrong. He continued to excel academically, too. Jamie, my younger brother, also continued to do very well in sports at the middle school level, and his grades were good.

When my dad was in a good mood, he was still great and fun to be around. There were times when my dad would go out and get my brothers and I chocolate chip cookies and potato chips. I think this was his way of trying to connect. I remember watching the NBA finals with my older brother and my dad, and the fact that I actually spoke with my dad during the game. It was the first time in several months that I said more than a few words to him.

My mom didn't want to be around my dad anymore and I couldn't blame her for it. After all those fights, we still ate together, but there was definitely a wall between my parents. I just wanted my dad to leave. At home I had to hear them fighting and at school I was bullied—there was no longer any refuge for me. I hated life more than ever. I became even more lonely and depressed.

By the time I got to my sophomore year, I didn't have any friends at school. I did everything by myself and still stuttered severely. In my freshman year, I had played on the basketball team, but then I started getting failing grades. I wasn't allowed to play until I brought my grades up, which never happened in ninth grade. For my sophomore year, I decided I wouldn't be involved in any sports so I could focus solely on my grades. I didn't want to go through the possibility of being academically ineligible again and possibly being taunted about my poor grades.

I had all the same subjects I had taken my freshman year: English, science, history, math, and physical education. I also had driver's education. I again went to my teachers at the beginning of the school year and asked them not to call on me if possible. That worked for several of my classes like English, science, and history, but not for French, math, or driver's education. My French teacher still called on me. As always, I didn't mind being called on in math class because I was still a wiz with numbers. That was the class where people focused on my abilities rather than on my severe disability. I was surprised and relieved that my classmates in this new math class were very patient with me.

Many of the students in my classes knew each other so they would hang out together. They could have known each other from the previous year, through social functions, or through a club or sport. I always felt left out. I didn't know what to do to be accepted by others. I was way too afraid to approach people in my classes and introduce myself. That was too risky for me. I wanted so much to have the courage to introduce myself to others, but the fear of stuttering made me feel like that was an impossible feat. I sat quietly in my classes and didn't say a word unless I was called upon.

It wasn't how I pictured high school to be, especially during my eighth-grade year when my stutter mysteriously vanished. I had watched my brother Jonathan go through high school involved in sports and going to social events, so I thought that was available for me as well. But I couldn't get past my stutter or my fear of it. While my classmates and other students in my high school went to dances, football games, basketball games, movies, dates, or just to a friend's house, I was at home in my bedroom looking at baseball cards, watching television, listening to my parents fight, or, on occasion, hanging out with my neighborhood friends. I thought, "This is my life and there is nothing I can do about it."

After a while, I got very tired of being by myself. I had to find something to do with my time. I could have turned to drugs or alcohol, but I watched what alcohol did to my dad and I didn't want any part of that, so I kept looking. Then

I found it. I turned my attention to food. Food became my friend. Every day after school during my sophomore year, I would go home and have two heaping bowls of butter pecan ice cream. I would follow that up with a box of chocolate chip cookies or Oreos, then I would have a one-pound bag of barbeque or sour cream & onion potato chips. I felt so good. I was satisfied and fulfilled for thirty minutes a day.

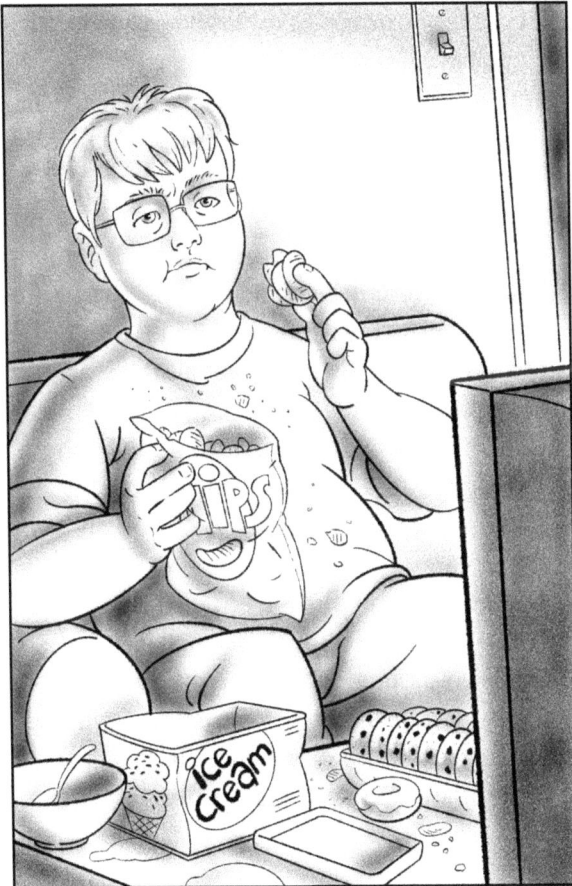

While I ate the food, I watched television with my younger brother. I really didn't care what he or anyone else thought about how much food I was consuming every day. The only thing that mattered to me was that for a short time during the day, I didn't have to talk to anyone. I didn't have to answer any questions. I got to do what I wanted to do. I got to eat what I wanted to eat. I got the chance to escape my problems.

I was eating five thousand calories a day. I was eating my parents out of house and home. I knew it was unhealthy, but I was so desperate for relief, I couldn't help it. I would gorge myself and then go back to being sad, lonely, depressed, and frustrated because I didn't have anyone to talk to. I started gaining a lot of weight and still couldn't speak without stuttering. Eating was my only outlet.

My parents were talking to each other even less. I thought they would get divorced but my dad kept living with us.

I couldn't talk with my parents about how I was feeling because they were so bogged down with their own issues. I didn't feel like I could talk to my neighborhood friends, either. They never asked how I was doing. All I knew was that eating made me feel good. It made me forget all the pain and frustration in my life for a while.

As bad as things were for me during my sophomore year, I did discover one bright spot: my driver's education class. My teacher's name was Mr. Hubbard. He was one funny guy, and also a very caring and loving person. I would go to his class and he would be standing outside of the classroom greeting all of the students who knew him. He seemed to know so many of them personally. I assumed they were all driver's ed students, then I remembered him sharing with our class that he was also one of the assistant football coaches. It made sense that so many students knew him. He was really beloved among the student body.

He told us, "Don't sweat this class. This will be your easy class." And he was right. But he also said, "If I catch you cheating in my class, you will fail the semester. I don't care what the administration says—that is my policy. So don't cheat." He was very straight with us.

Mr. Hubbard was a very approachable guy. Many of my classmates went up to him after class just to talk and a lot of football players stopped to check in with him. However, it took me several weeks before I spoke with Mr. Hubbard after class. I was scared that he was going to be like every other teacher I had who didn't seem to care, that he would only be interested in grades. But I discovered that Mr. Hubbard was much more concerned with people. He was the first teacher who ever listened to me and didn't interrupt regardless of how badly I stuttered. Sometimes, it would take me three minutes just to get out a word or a sentence, and he was right there with me, patiently listening. I knew for at least one period per week that I was going to be listened to, respected, appreciated, and loved. I knew that no one in that class was going to laugh at me because Mr. Hubbard wouldn't stand for it. I was able to understand why he was loved and admired by so many people.

I was sad when my class ended. He let all of us know that if we ever needed anything, his door was always open. I was stunned. I couldn't believe I knew a teacher who was interested in me and not just my grades. Even though I never took him up on the offer to speak with him about my problems, it was a big deal to me that he offered.

It wasn't long after the semester ended that Mr. Hubbard was named the new head football coach at Wissahickon, which seemed to make a lot of people very happy. He was pretty young at the time to get a head-coaching job. I believe he was twenty-eight years old. When I saw him in the hallway one day, I congratulated him and said, "Maybe I'll come and try out for the football team."

He replied, "I would love that, Billy."

Being around Mr. Hubbard was inspiring. He always had a smile on his face and he cared about everyone. It's such a simple thing yet many find it very difficult to accomplish.

12

The Best Year

There I was approaching the end of my sophomore year and I had gained fifty-five pounds. Deciding not to play sports was a bad move for me. Now, not only were people laughing at me for stuttering, they were also laughing at me for being overweight. I looked like I had breasts. Needless to say, it wasn't very becoming. I also had a learning disability. I had poor grades and was failing 80% of my classes in the first two years of high school. I had family problems, no friends, and still stuttered severely. I was committed to doing everything alone, and it made me miserable. I hated my life. I didn't want to be at home or school. I was at the lowest point in my life and didn't know what to do. I had reached a crossroads and I needed to find a clear path for myself. I just wasn't sure what that was going to be.

At the end of my sophomore year, I had to attend an assembly. Several upperclassmen spoke, including a junior I knew. His name was Bruce Christopher and he was the junior class president. I decided I would give him my full attention. As he spoke, one statement really stuck with me. He said, "Go make next year the best year of your life!" I decided in that moment that I had been sad, lonely, frustrated, and depressed long enough, and I was going to do something about it.

I decided to go out for the football team. The first thing I did was tell Coach Hubbard my plan. He thanked me for letting him know, and told me there would be training over the summer he thought I ought to attend. I said I would. Before I could get to this training, though, I had to attend summer school for several classes. That was something else I was tired of doing—failing classes and attending summer school. I had to go after ninth grade as well. I didn't like it, but I knew if I did the right work and studied, I wouldn't have to go back.

During summer school, I ran into a guy I knew named Bob Morehouse. He asked me, "Bill, when are you going to start coming to the training sessions?" I said, "I didn't know that they had started."

Actually, that wasn't the case. As usual, I just didn't want to confront my fears of socializing and speaking with other people that might laugh at my stutter. Then I thought about the commitment I had made to myself to turn my life around and thought, "I am done having those feelings. I am just going to be courageous and face my fear of stuttering as best as I can."

The next day I decided to go to the training program Coach Hubbard and his staff were offering. I had about a mile-and-a-half walk to the training, which began at 6:30 p.m. I was nervous because up until that point in my high school career, I had never done anything socially, and I hadn't participated in sports in two years. I was also very concerned, as always, that my teammates were going to laugh at my stutter. I felt almost as nervous as I did before my oral presentation in history class. My heart was racing and sweat was pouring down my face. I walked the mile-and-a-half and reached the high school fifteen minutes early. I nearly talked myself out of going in and introducing myself, but then I reminded myself again of how tired I was of being frustrated and alone.

The summer training program was being held in our domed gymnasium. I walked down the steps and the first person to see me was Coach Hubbard. He said, "Billy! Good to see you! Go introduce yourself to the other people who are here tonight." I noticed how much worry was building up inside of me. I couldn't believe I was actually there and that I was going to introduce myself.

Before I could introduce myself, several seniors approached me. "I'm Bruce," one said.

"I'm Drew," said another.

"I'm Brian."

"I'm Mark."

"I'm Tony. What's your name?"

I thought to myself, "Oh no. I am actually going to have to say my name. I hope they don't laugh at me too much. Please, God, just this once, let me say my name without stuttering. If I can say my name fluently, these seniors will accept me."

I took a deep breath and said, "My name is B-b-b-b-b-b-b-b-b-b-b-b-b-b-b-b-b-b-b-b-b-b-b-b-b-b-b-b-b-b-b-b-b-b-b-b-b-b-b-b-b-b-b-b-um-um-um-um-um-um-um-um-um-um-um-um-um-um-um-um-um my n-n-n-n-n-n-n-n-n-ame i-i-i-is B-b-b-b-b-b-b-i-i-i-i-i-i-i-i-i-l-l-l-l-l-l-l-l-l. My name is Bill." It took me about forty-five seconds to get my first name out. Looking at me you would have thought I had just run a marathon because sweat was pouring down my face and my t-shirt was nearly soaked.

I was waiting for the seniors to laugh at me. When I said my name, they all made eye contact with me, which was something I wasn't used to. I never made eye contact with anyone. I was always too afraid of the reaction I would get. When I finally got my name out, they all greeted me in a variety of friendly ways. One said, "Bill, it's nice to meet you. Thank you for coming out." I was shocked. It was the first time in my high school career that no one laughed at my stuttering. I couldn't believe it.

Inside I thought, "What a miracle. I might actually have a chance at having friends." But I didn't want to push it. After meeting these seniors, I met other people on the team, and they were very kind to me, too. I wondered where they all had been during my first two years of high school. It would have been nice to have known them then as well.

Coach Hubbard brought everyone together and had a few words for the new people. Then we got to stretching and doing some football exercises. I thought for sure that once I began doing the football exercises I would get laughed at. I hadn't done many of the exercises in a couple years, and I was sixty pounds lighter then. One of the exercises we had to do involved getting into a four-point stance. I was having trouble keeping my balance and not crawling on my knees. I was weak, out of shape and out of breath. Throughout all of the exercises, and especially this one, no one laughed at me. Instead, people were cheering me on, saying, "Come on, Billy! You can do this!" I was stunned by my teammates' generosity toward me.

At the end of the night, those same seniors who had introduced themselves came up to me and one of them said, "Way to go, Bill! Will we see you tomorrow?" I said yes, and then one of the team captains, Bruce Christopher, asked me if he could give me a ride home. I enthusiastically accepted. He was the same person who, just a few months before, as junior class president, said, "Go make next year the best year of your life." From the conversation on the ride home, I remember how great I felt having someone care about me. I left so excited that night because there was a good chance I was going to make new friends who I could hang out with and who would be there when I needed them. That was what I had wanted for so long.

Everything seemed to get a lot better; even going to summer school the next day and for the few weeks that were left. I couldn't wait to go back to the summer training program. By no means was I in good shape, but I attended the program, made great strides, and laughed and joked around with my teammates. I had never before had an opportunity to "let my hair down" so to speak. I had always kept my guard up, waiting for someone to laugh at me, but that was beginning to change.

There was one summer training session that will always stick out in my mind. We all had to run a half-mile around the track. Coach Hubbard separated us by class. The seniors went first, then the juniors, and finally the sophomores. The seniors on the team were a very close-knit group and they finished up pretty quickly. Then the juniors ran. That was my group.

I waited for Coach Hubbard to blow his whistle so the run could begin. I was very nervous because even though I had been attending all of the sessions, I had never run more than one hundred meters at a time. Now I would have to cover eight hundred meters. I figured I would just focus on doing the best I could. Coach Hubbard blew his whistle and we were off. I started off quickly, thinking I could keep up the pace of my fellow juniors. That wasn't the case. After the first hundred meters, I was huffing and puffing as I watched my teammates get way ahead of me. After two hundred meters, I was ready to quit.

I was about to stop when I noticed one of the team captains sprinting across the football field. He ran over to me and said, "Billy, I'm going to run the last half with you. We're gonna do this together." It was Bruce Christopher. Every step of the way he said, "Come on, Billy. Come on, Billy. You can do this." As we got closer and closer to the finish line, I noticed my teammates were rooting us on. About a hundred meters out, Bruce turned to me and said, "Billy, we're going to sprint through that finish line." I had never run so hard in my life, and I made it to the finish line. All of my teammates came up to me and said, "Way to go, Bill," shaking my hand or patting me on the back. I looked at Coach Hubbard, and he looked very proud of me.

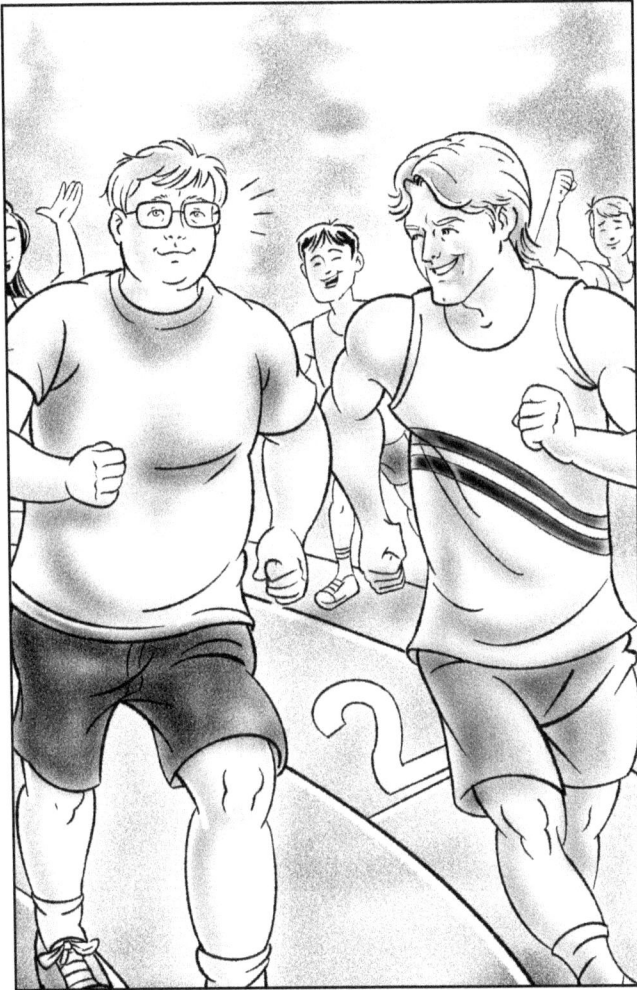

When I crossed that finish line, it was like all the times I said I couldn't do it were behind me. I decided in that moment that I would never give up again. I didn't care what problems might arise in my life. I learned so much over that summer about things that weren't taught in class. I learned the importance of being dedicated, determined, disciplined, and persistent. I learned to persevere through adversity. I learned that I could achieve much more with a team than as an individual. I went back for my junior year with a whole new outlook on my life. I had goals and I was going to achieve them.

I also created a number of new friendships, including all of those seniors who had introduced themselves on the first day I attended the summer training camp. After camp, we had a week off, and then the real football camp began. When football began, I kept getting sick and dizzy. Coach Hubbard told me I would be better off as a manager or keeping the statistics, so that's what I did. My teammates didn't seem to mind. They actually liked having me around. Despite not participating in the football drills, I still went to both practices every day. I loved being around people who wanted me to be there and wanted to be my friends. That was so much the opposite of my experience in school so far.

I started creating friendships with other people on the team, including Andy and Derek, who were in my class. They were always very upbeat. Andy liked to joke around with me about my stutter, but I didn't mind. In fact, I appreciated it because I knew he was attempting to bring some lightness to a situation that had always been so dark and painful for me. He liked finishing my sentences for me. At first, it really bothered me and he would apologize, but then I got used to it and would let him finish them. That was a first for me. Because of his good nature and the knowledge that he had my best interests at heart, I was able to set my pride down, stop taking myself so seriously, and let him help me. This was a huge step forward. I had always taken my stutter so seriously and had been unwilling to let anyone help me. Andy showed me that stuttering had far less power over me once I learned to laugh at it.

When football camp ended, it was time to start my junior year of high school. As I said, I had goals and I was going to achieve them. My goal entering my junior year was to get no grade lower than a C. Judging by my past performance, there was no evidence I could do that. I had failed miserably my first two years. But I was committed to it and now I had supportive people in my life who were willing to stand by me in the pursuit of my goal. What I ended up doing was reaching out to my principal, guidance counselor, teachers, and friends from the football team and asking them to support me. To my surprise, everyone was willing to help. For the first time in my life, I was actually excited to go to school. I was still very nervous and worried but now I had friends who were willing to be there and stick up for me. That was a great feeling. I looked forward to seeing them every day. Many of them weren't in my classes, but I would run into them in the hallways. They always smiled and greeted me with, "Hey, Billy." That became the name they called me. I didn't mind. I just liked that people were smiling at me and interested in knowing me. Anytime I ran into Coach Hubbard, he seemed to be in a good mood. He always smiled and asked me, "How you doin', Billy?"

My classes were challenging. Besides the four main subjects, I also had business, law, and accounting. Many of my classmates liked my accounting teacher. His name was Mr. Roberts. He was in his mid-twenties. Like Mr. Hubbard, he was a coach, but for basketball and lacrosse. He called me Billy, too.

Football practice started right after school. I went to every practice and helped out with the equipment. I think the coaches and players appreciated that I was out there with them. After practice, my friend Bruce would usually offer me a ride home; if not, sometimes I would just walk the mile or so. My mom must have seen a difference in me. I wasn't spending all my time emptying the refrigerator anymore. When dinner was over, without fail, I went up to my room and studied.

By that time, my parents had divorced. I lived with my mom and younger brother. My older brother, Jonathan, was now a sophomore at the University of Pennsylvania and living on campus. I knew my mom was struggling financially but she always managed to take care of our basic needs—and we always got presents on Christmas. My dad rarely showed up and I refused to speak with him when he did. I was still really angry with him even though I didn't want to be. I wanted to love my father, and I wanted him to love me. In a way, I should be grateful that my father showed me what can happen when, instead of asking for help, you try to avoid your problems and become more and more lonely, frustrated, and angry. It cost him his marriage and, for many years, the love of his children. I had been trying to escape my problems with food, and my father used alcohol. Maybe if my dad had asked for help sooner, things would have been different for him and my mom.

My dad attempted to my buy my love by giving me a television in my sophomore year. Then he gave me a check for several hundred dollars in my junior year. But what I really wanted was for him to apologize to my mom and to take full responsibility for his actions and the impact they'd had on my younger brother and me. But he never did. I accepted the television and money, but I still refused to talk to him, which saddened my brothers and grandmother as well as my dad.

During that time, I wasn't ready to forgive my dad and move on. I was determined not to talk with him, at least through high school. I just didn't want to have anything to do with him. When he called, I told my mom to say I wasn't there. As long as I had my mom, that's all that mattered to me.

I also relied on my new friends from the football team. I wasn't much of a talker, but I did enjoy being around them at football practice, at games and at school. I still wasn't attending any social events like dances. When I wasn't studying or at school or a football game, I spent my time watching television and eating. My eating wasn't as out of control as it had been my sophomore year, but I still used food as therapy. Fortunately, I only allowed myself smaller portions of my dietary staples—ice cream, cookies, and potato chips.

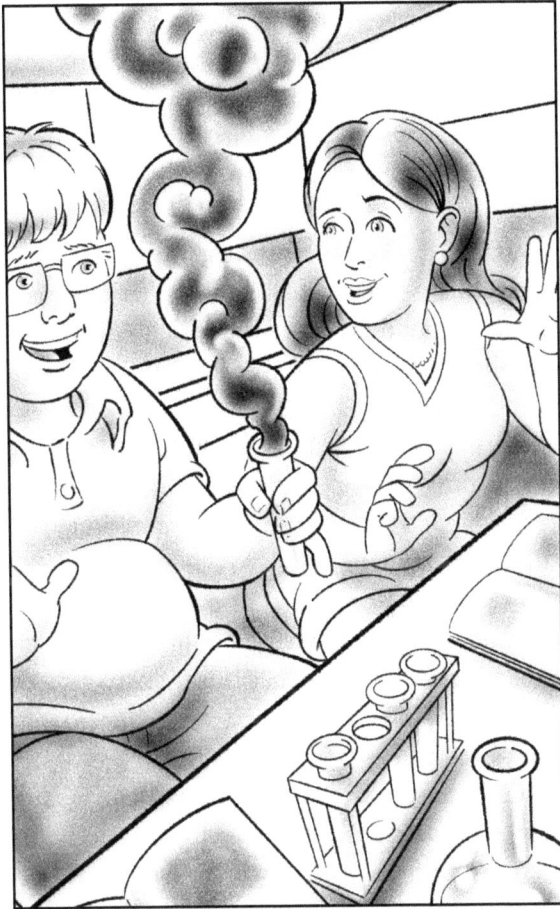

One of the classes I came to enjoy was chemistry. What made chemistry so interesting was that my teacher didn't seat us alphabetically. I ended up sitting next to a girl I had often passed by in the halls, Alyssa. I had never spoken to her because, as always, I was afraid she would laugh at me. This was not an irrational fear; it was simply my experience. When I stuttered, people laughed. When I finally got the nerve up to talk to her, I was happily surprised to see that she didn't laugh; she actually listened to me. Sometimes it would take me several minutes to say a sentence and she would wait for me to say it. That meant a lot to me.

Up until my junior year, I hadn't had many interactions with girls, so our short conversations were major events for me. After all, I usually avoided girls. It was somehow much worse for girls to laugh at me than for other guys to laugh at me.

After our first few conversations, Alyssa said hello to me when she saw me between classes. I couldn't believe it. I felt like I had a new friend, and a female friend at that. The more I spoke with her, the more comfortable I became with her and my other classmates that sat near me.

My chemistry teacher noticed what was happening, too, and started calling on me in class. I didn't mind because I studied every day, so I knew most of the answers to his questions. I still wasn't secure enough to raise my hand on my own, but it was a step in the right direction. Now I had not only my football friends, but also new friends in my other classes. As my self-esteem and self-confidence improved, and I had people who were there for me, the bullying and teasing stopped.

Studying every day and having the support of my teachers, guidance counselor, principal, and friends paid off. My grades improved dramatically. I was now receiving A's and B's. I was so proud of myself. My team was proud of me, too, and so was my mom. I had never gotten A's or B's in high school before. It was a thrilling experience. It made me realize that if I continued to work hard, be disciplined, and accept the support of my team, I could achieve anything I wanted in life. I reached my goal of not getting a grade lower than C for the entire year. What made the biggest difference for me was stepping beyond my fear and getting involved in my school. I wasn't going to allow myself to hide anymore. I had as much to offer as anyone else.

13

200 Pounds

Being on the football team my junior year was an experience I will always remember. Our team didn't win many games, but no one ever pointed fingers at each other. Coach Hubbard made it clear that we won and lost as a team. The last game of the year was also the last football game that most of the seniors were going to play. It was a hard-fought game on Thanksgiving, and we won over our rivals, Upper Dublin, with a score of 7-6. The seniors lifted Coach Hubbard in the air. When we got back to our locker room, a lot of tears were shed among my teammates. I found myself crying as well. Even though I wasn't playing, I had been very close to the team for nearly six months. I knew what it was like to be loved by the coaching staff as well as the players, and I loved them, too.

We had a banquet at the end of football season. My friend Bruce gave me a ride. During the banquet, the coaches gave out the team awards. I got a certificate for being on the team. It was a lot of fun. Coach Hubbard had been tough and emotional. He had a big heart and loved us all. At the time, it was the most fulfilling experience of my life.

I still saw many of the players from the football team around school; some of them were in my classes as well. After football season, I decided to go out for indoor track. Someone had suggested it might be fun for me, and he was right. It turned out to be a good outlet. Though not very glamorous, it got me out of my house and, more importantly, out of my own head. I had learned in a big way from my experience with the football team that being around other people was good for me.

There were a lot of Saturday track meets where the best runners on the team would compete in their respective events. There were also a few meets in which I got to participate against another team. I chose the shot-put event. There were three other shot-putters. Mick Pernas was the best. He was a junior as well. The other two were Willard and Joe, both sophomores. Even though Mick was the best, he was laid back and didn't have a big ego. All of us got along very well and cheered each other on. Joe had just arrived from Baltimore and didn't really know anyone except Bruce from the football team because their parents were friends. Bruce asked me if I would be Joe's friend and I said, "Of course!" If anyone knew what it was like to be alone, it was me. Joe and I quickly became good friends. Although he was a year younger than me, he was very smart, especially when it came to math.

Besides the track team, I also started socializing a bit. Bruce invited me to go to a few of our school's basketball games; typically, the ones away from home. He picked me up, along with his girlfriend at the time, and we met up with some of the other people I knew from the football team—the students who had introduced themselves to me so kindly the first time I had attended summer training six months earlier. I really enjoyed hanging out with Bruce and my other friends. I couldn't believe there was actually another way to live my life. And all of it was possible just because I had taken the risk of stepping beyond my fear and going to the summer training program. I had been scared to death that everyone would laugh at me, and there I was, six months later, sitting at a basketball game with a bunch of new friends who wanted me to be there. I looked around the gymnasium at the fans, the players on both teams, and my friends' bright faces and thought, "This is what it is like to live, be involved, have fun, and be fulfilled. I want this feeling to last as long as possible."

When basketball season ended, my friends headed to their respective spring sports—baseball or lacrosse. I didn't mind because I went out for the spring track team. The difference between the winter and spring teams were the number of people and coaches. There were more coaches for spring and more team members as well.

This time, I threw the discus as well as the shot put. I remember watching the 1984 Olympics and thinking how cool both of those events looked. I decided then and there to try it myself. There was a coach for each discipline—one for the sprints and hurdles, another for the jumps and pole vault, and a third, my coach, for the weight events. His name was Mr. Richardson. He had just stepped down as the head football coach within the last year. Ironically, I knew him because he had been my third-grade physical education teacher. I hadn't seen him since then. He looked about the same, only a bit older. He remembered who I was, but he wasn't someone who played favorites.

In addition to the three people I had gotten to know from winter track, there were now another four or five people participating in the weight events. There was Andy, who I knew from the football team, and Francis, an exchange student from Italy. Francis would always get mad when anyone spat around him. He would yell, "Don't spit!" I guess it grossed him out, or it was more offensive in Italy. He was the spit police of the team.

There was a great camaraderie among my teammates in the weight events. We pushed each other, and Mr. Richardson pushed all of us. We worked out with weights twice a week and he had us run a couple of times a week, too. I didn't like to do either of these tasks, especially the running part, because I was still obese. One day, about a month into track season, Mr. Richardson had us run up and down the bleachers. I was the last one done, and I was exhausted. Afterwards, he took me aside and said, "Billy, you need to lose some weight if you want to improve in your events. You could be two hundred pounds by the end of the track season."

I took his words to heart, mainly because I liked him so much. He was tough, but he cared. So I decided that on Friday, March 29, 1985, I would start my diet. At the time, I weighed two hundred thirty-three pounds and had a forty-four-inch waist. I knew the first weeks were going to be the hardest because the first week was my brother's birthday, which meant cake and ice cream, both of which I loved. The following week happened to be Easter, which meant chocolate, which I also loved. When I got home that day and told my mom and younger brother I was going on a diet, they laughed. My brother said, "Bill, you're gonna fail. You'll go on a diet for a few days or a week and then go back to eating all the junk food you can get your hands on." I realized from this reaction that I had created the impression with my family that I didn't follow through on my promises. I made a commitment to myself to change that.

My younger brother's birthday was on April 2. I did have a little piece of cake but that was all. After that piece, I decided to give up all junk food, which included cake, cookies, ice cream, candy, crackers, pretzels, potato chips, Doritos, and pizza—any food that wasn't a fruit, vegetable, or meat.

The week of Easter was the hardest seven days of my life. My younger brother tempted me with chocolate the entire time as well as on Easter, but I didn't cave. When my friends who ate with me found out I was on a diet, they also tried to tempt me with cakes, cookies, and ice cream. They laughed and said, "Bill, doesn't this look so good? I know you want some."

I said, "It does look good, but not for me, because I'm on a diet."

That shut them right up. I used my willpower to get through the first two weeks. I remember suffering from headaches as my body tried to adjust to my new way of eating. I thought if I could make it through those two weeks, I could make it through anything. And I was right.

I did make it through the first two weeks without eating any sweets or junk food other than that little piece of cake on my brother's birthday. My friends who ate lunch with me realized how serious I was, stopped tempting me with sweets, and began to encourage me. They became my biggest supporters.

Every day after track practice was over, I ran about eight times around the fence that surrounded our main track. I calculated that it was three to four miles. When I first started, I was very slow. It took me about sixteen minutes per mile. That was my starting point. After most people left, I was still running, or doing a very slow jog. When I jogged after practice, I always ran into at least one of my friends who would cheer me on with comments like, "Come on, Billy! You can do it!" Every time I felt like stopping, their words repeated in my mind and encouraged me to keep going.

I weighed in on an electronic scale owned by Mr. Doyleson, an athletic trainer who also happened to be my biology teacher during my sophomore year. Everyone called him Guy. He stayed on my back a lot, but I knew it was because he really cared. Every week, I got weighed in. After a month, I had lost fourteen pounds. I couldn't believe it. I still had another nineteen pounds to go so my weight loss wasn't that noticeable yet, but I was doing well and accomplishing my goals. I was still studying every day and doing well in my classes, too. I had friends to hang out with at lunch and friends on the track team. I wasn't much for talking but I listened a lot. I shared a lot of laughs. I was improving in my events. My self-esteem and self-confidence also continued to improve dramatically.

I was still running every day after track practice, even when I didn't want to run. There were days I wanted to blow it off because it was raining, or cold, or hot, or my legs were sore, or I had cramps, or I just didn't feel like it. But then I thought to myself, "If I don't run, I am not going to reach my goal of two hundred pounds by the end of track season. If I don't run, how am I going to get in better shape? How am I going to improve in my events? I have to run even if I don't want to because if I do, I will lose the weight I want, have the body I want, and be in the best shape of my life." I just kept my goal in mind and focused on that.

There were times when I was running alone on an empty track and I really had to push myself and dig deep to complete the three miles. Sometimes the pain from the cramps in my stomach made me want to stop, but I always remembered a trick my older brother, Jonathan, told me he used for this problem. It was not advice that would get rid of the pain, unfortunately. He told me to bite my lip to take my focus off of my cramp! It sounded crazy at first but it worked every time. When no one was around, I had to encourage myself. I talked to myself using the same language my friends did: "Come on, Billy! You can do this! You can make it! Just keep pushing yourself." I had never pushed myself as hard as I did when I was running laps and losing weight. After two months, I had lost a total of twenty-seven pounds. I fell short of my weight goal of two hundred, but that didn't matter because I was proud of what I had accomplished; and I wasn't stopping. I was going to keep running and losing weight over the summer.

By the end of track season, I was running a mile in twelve minutes instead of sixteen. I also had to go out and buy smaller pants. My teachers and friends from the football team started noticing my weight loss and let me know they were proud of me. I couldn't believe the difference in my life that getting involved in my school's activities had made.

My junior year of high school was about to end. By the summer, I really started to enjoy jogging. Sometimes I would run twice a day even if the temperature soared into the nineties. It didn't matter to me.

At the end of June 1985, I went back to the summer training program for the football team, except now I was a senior. I made a commitment to myself to go to every session and get a t-shirt with "I paid the price" printed on it. It was an honor to get one of those shirts because not everyone attended every session. I still struggled with some of the football exercises, but my teammates rooted me on anyway. I saw some of my friends who graduated, too. Sometimes Bruce and I would run together. I also got to see some other friends who came and worked out in the weight room. It was good to see them, and they still inspired me.

Many of my fellow teammates worked. I didn't. It didn't even cross my mind to get a job. My friends cut lawns or worked in movie theaters. My only focus was to lose weight and get in the best shape possible so I could give football camp another shot.

I attended all of the summer training sessions and received the "I paid the price" t-shirt I wanted. I wore that shirt with pride. I lost another fourteen pounds for a total of forty-one pounds by the time football camp try-outs began. I felt like I was in good shape and I was ready to give it a shot. The first day of camp, we got our equipment and there was no hitting. Then came the next day. I was really nervous because I wasn't sure how all the running I did was going to help me on the football field. When we started hitting, I realized I didn't like it at all. I just wasn't used to it. I was still getting sick and feeling dizzy from the summer sun. I sat out the next few practices. One night, my brother, Jonathan, asked me how football camp was going. I said, "I'm feeling dizzy and getting sick."

He replied, "Bill, maybe you should consider the possibility that football is not for you. I think it's great that you lost all the weight you did and have gotten in good shape, but that's only part of playing football. There is no shame in not playing. Just think about it."

The more I thought about it, the more I realized he was right. I really didn't like getting hit. In fact, I was afraid to get hit hard. I knew the difficult part would be telling Coach Hubbard that I wasn't going to play football, and why.

I lived about a mile-and-a-half from the high school. We had two practices a day in the afternoon and evening, so I jogged up to the school in the morning. Coach Hubbard was there. He was always there, even at one in the morning. He loved coaching. I was nervous about speaking with him. When I got to my high school, I knocked on the door. He walked down the hallway and said, "Hi, Billy! What can I do for you?"

I said, "I need to talk with you."

We walked into his office and sat down. I said, "Mr. Hubbard, I'm feeling sick and dizzy and don't think I can make it through camp."

I thought that was a really good reason. I didn't want to tell him the real reason was that I couldn't take a hit. But he didn't buy it. He knew that there was something more, so he pressed me. I finally broke down and said, "I'm afraid to take a hard hit. That's why. I'm not going to be able to make it through camp." I was so ashamed, I just started crying, and that only made me feel more shameful.

Coach Hubbard said, "Bill, it takes a lot of courage to say that. I have a tremendous amount of respect for you. I knew this day was coming; I just wasn't sure when."

I was shocked when Mr. Hubbard started crying, too. I still am. It's so rare to find a teacher that feels so deeply for his students. It's hard to find a *friend* like that. He said, "What are you going to do now? Do you still want to be on the team to do the stats or be a manager?"

When I didn't answer, he said, "I'll leave that up to you,

Bill. You're going to have to start making your own decisions and this will be one of them."

As I got ready to leave, Coach Hubbard surprised me again by giving me a hug and saying, "Billy, I love you."

After I left, I walked home crying the whole way. I was sad about the loss of my dream of playing football, but also very touched by Coach Hubbard's compassion for me. I also realized that while I had been avoiding my own father, Coach Hubbard had in some way become like a father to me. He was the kind that called me courageous for admitting my fear. He was proud of me and he loved me. It really made a difference to have a father figure like Coach Hubbard in my life.

By the time I arrived home, all of my tears were gone. That was good, because I didn't want my younger brother to see that I was upset. He was on the couch with his homework in his lap. I went to my room and got in bed. As I thought about it more, I realized that my dream was not really to play football; it was to have friends, camaraderie, and the feeling of being part of a team. I decided to stay on the team and keep the stats.

The next problem I had was what to tell my friends on the team when they asked why I wasn't practicing. I was afraid they would lose respect for me if I told them the real reason, so I just said it was due to being sick and dizzy. They seemed to accept that. They asked me if I was going to stay on the team and keep the stats again and I said yes. They were happy about my decision. I let Coach Hubbard know and he was happy, too. Having the support of the coaches and my teammates went a long way to soothe the disappointment of not being able to play. I still attended every afternoon and evening practice throughout football camp and ate my meals with my teammates. It was a lot of fun, without the hitting!

After football camp, it was on to my senior year of high school. I was actually excited about it. I was thrilled that girls from my class were speaking to me. Girls saying hello and smiling at me took some getting used to, but that was an adjustment I was very happy to make. My classmates, friends, and administrators complimented me on my weight loss. At the beginning of the year, a lot of people asked me how many pounds I had dropped.

My answer was always, "I have lost fifty-two pounds and I feel great!" Having the respect and admiration of my friends and classmates was becoming my new normal, and after a lifetime of the polar opposite, it felt amazing. I also felt good because of my running, and because I wasn't eating foods that made me feel tired.

Previously, I had taken classes just to fill my schedule and get through the day. Now that I had some self-confidence, I scheduled classes with people I enjoyed being around. In addition to learning, classes were now an opportunity to develop friendships and have fun. I challenged myself a bit by taking a few college-prep classes, including economics. I had the same economics teacher as my sophomore year. He was more intense in this class, but I didn't mind. Our football team was better than it had been the previous year. We didn't have a winning record, but we didn't lose as many games as the year before. Coach Hubbard was one of the hardest workers I had ever met in my life. He would arrive at school every day at 7:00 a.m., work all day, then watch football films until 1:00 a.m. He rarely took a break. I would often run at night and see a solitary light on in the high school. Everyone knew it was Coach Hubbard's light. While the other teachers were home relaxing, he was obsessing about how he could help his students. He was as kind to everyone as he had been to me. He loved sharing in their personal triumphs and revel in their accomplishments right along with them. He would also get upset when players or students shared bad news. He was always right there for us, regardless of the situation. That was the main reason he was so beloved among students.

Coach Hubbard could be very intense when he had to be

but very loving, too. He said his door was always open for the football players and really anyone who wanted to speak with him. I spent a lot of time talking with him about all kinds of things, in his office or when he gave me rides home. He always made time for me and seemed genuinely interested in getting updates on my progress. He was one of the most encouraging, inspiring, and empowering people I had ever met in my life.

He was also a very funny guy, cracking jokes at football practice and coming up with silly phrases. He had us all cracking up. And he had a great laugh. The other coaches were funny, too. One of them was Mr. Lattice. He told us that when we got headaches, we should just pretend to rake our hands over our eyes and that would get rid of them. I tried it to amuse him. I was happy to find a place at my school where I felt comfortable to be myself.

I enjoyed being the stats person again. I got to watch games from the press box. On colder nights, it was nice because I didn't have to freeze my butt off. I knew that what I was doing was very helpful for the team. I liked everything about Friday nights: the beat of the drums from our school band, all the fans and fellow schoolmates who came out to support the team, and the cheerleaders. I liked Coach Hubbard's pep talks. Some were longer than others but they all usually ended with him telling us how much he loved us.

Being on the sidelines was fun, too. It was great to hang out and watch my teammates work together to win a game and share some laughs with them. After the games were over, it was back to the locker room for a post-game meeting with Coach Hubbard and the other coaches. Losses were hard to take. When we won, everyone was on a high, and when we lost, the mood was somber.

After football season was over, it was on to indoor track. When my track coach saw me, he said, "Bill, you look like a high jumper or a hurdler, not a shot-putter!" I took that as a compliment. I felt like I was finally in the shape I needed to be in for the running I had to do in the winter. There was a new shot-putter on the team that year named Stan Amica. His older brother held the school record in the shot put. Stan looked like he could move an eighteen-wheeler truck by himself. He was about five feet, eleven inches and one hundred and eighty-five pounds of muscle. He pushed all of us to develop a stronger work ethic. His throws in the shot put were a good five to six feet further than that of our best shot-putter the year before, my friend Mick. Our group of five worked out two to three times a week. It didn't take long for us all to build great relationships with one another. We pushed each other in the weight room, in throwing the shot put, and in the running we did. We got along very well.

Winter track was all about the Saturday meets. That's where the best of the best from each high school got together and tested their talent to win in events ranging from sprints to jumps, to hurdles, to weight events. In my two years of track, I never participated in the Saturday meets. Stan Amica was our shot-put representative. He did very well. His throws were consistently over fifty feet. He was very competitive and wanted to win every meet. He got frustrated and annoyed when he didn't win.

I could have attended the Saturday meets during the winter, but I didn't. I stayed home and watched television or went for a run. Sometimes after track practice, I would run three miles on our indoor track, which at times got very boring. Seeing the same things over and over again can get to you. Still, running became a great outlet for me. I often imagined I was running away from what I didn't want anymore and toward what I did. When a particularly upsetting memory crossed my mind, I found myself running faster, running farther from it, leaving it behind, and burning the memory right out of me.

14

Most Improved

During my senior year, I had to go to a specialty doctor. I found out that I had Klein Felter's Syndrome, which meant that I had an extra chromosome. Usually a man has one X and one Y chromosome in each cell, but I found out that I had an extra X chromosome (XXY). When my doctor explained what the extra chromosome was and the impact it would have on my health, I was actually relieved. Before I went to see the doctor, I was told I might have to get an operation. However, I saw an endocrinologist and was told that I only needed to get a shot of testosterone in my arm every two weeks.

The doctor told me Klein Felter's Syndrome was a possible cause for my stuttering and learning disability. Finding out there was possibly a physical reason for my problems was a revelation to me because of all the times I had blamed and condemned myself for not having the strength or skill to overcome them. I didn't do it to myself. My body did it. Knowing that as a younger child would have prevented a lot of self-criticism. I had bullied myself internally as much as anyone else had.

I also found out that I had a low testosterone level, which was why I looked so young for my age. I looked like a twelve-year-old kid during my senior year of high school. I didn't have any facial hair and had very little hair on my arms and legs. The medication would help me look closer to my age. I would grow more hair on my arms and legs and need to shave once a week or so. The medication would also help me feel sexual attraction, which I had never really felt before. Even with the medication, though, I was told I would never be able to have my own children. At eighteen years old, having children hadn't really crossed my mind yet, but it was important for me to know. I was too young to completely process this information. Lastly, I had to take the medication consistently so I wouldn't get osteoporosis.

Every two weeks, I made sure I went to my family doctor to get my shot. That part was easy but visiting the doctor's office wasn't. I still struggled when I attempted to say my name when checking in or talking to the nurse. Many times, they became impatient and asked me to just write my name down. In those instances, I felt very embarrassed. I actually started to consider changing my name to something without B's or D's so I wouldn't stutter so badly and so people wouldn't look at me like there was something wrong with me. All the while, I hoped that the shots would help me eventually lose my stutter forever.

The thing I noticed most after getting my first shot was the instant energy it gave me. I also began to grow facial hair and more hair on my legs, and I really started noticing women. I just didn't know what to do with all the sexual energy I had never felt before. I was still really shy and stuttered severely, so I did what was comfortable for me, which was to say very little and keep to myself.

My last semester of high school began with my friend, teacher, and athletic trainer, Guy Doyleson, suggesting that I try progressive relaxation to help my stutter. He told me it would put me in a hypnotic state. At this point, I was willing to try anything. Two to three times a week, I had a free period and went to see him. He explained that he would relax my whole body and then give me certain phrases to remember. One of my friends would sometimes come with me. The times that I was really willing to let go and put myself under, I was able to notice a difference in my speech.

Even as a senior, everything still revolved around my speech. My friends didn't care if I stuttered or not, but it still bothered me. I figured if I didn't stutter, I could be really confident and live my life to the fullest. Living to my highest potential with a very severe stutter wasn't a possibility in my mind. I still struggled at times with my speech and got very embarrassed. Everyone knew when I felt embarrassed because my face turned beet red. Blushing only added to the frustration of having no control over what my body did. The irony is, the only person who was really bothered by my stuttering was me. I couldn't get away from it and I wasn't willing to accept it. I must have wished and prayed a million times throughout my life that somehow my stutter would disappear and I could start living fully and be normal like everyone else.

My friends could tell that it really bothered me. One of them, Andy, was determined to bring lightness to the situation. I had a music class with him and one day, we had to do a skit together. He called me Porky Bill, as in the Porky Pig cartoon. But when I tried to stutter in the skit, I couldn't! The one time I really wanted to stutter, I suddenly spoke easily. But Andy was still successful in his attempt to make me take myself less seriously. He called me Porky Bill until I started laughing. He wouldn't let up until he could see I was enjoying myself.

Andy was one of the few people I allowed to finish my sentences for me. I once asked him why he kept doing it and he said, "Bill, I know how much you struggle with your stutter and I just want to ease some of your pain and help you out."

I was really touched by that. When Andy was with me, I knew he had my back and would finish the sentences I couldn't get out. He was the kind of person who put everyone at ease. He was a terror on the football field but the nicest, funniest guy you could ever meet otherwise.

I was excited about spring track my senior year of high school. The same people from the previous year came back, with some new additions. The shot-putters, discus throwers, and javelin throwers—also known as the weight throwers—all got a new coach. Coach Richardson stepped down from his role. Our new coach was Jon Amica, the giant who held the school record in the shot put. His best throw was fifty-five feet and four inches, a tremendous throw by any standard. The person to come closest to beating his record was his younger brother, Stan, who was a junior on the team this year. Jon was about twenty-eight years old. He wasn't a big believer in running like Coach Richardson was. He was all about weight-lifting. Our team lifted together three times a week, every week, even weeks when we had two track meets. We also spent a lot of time working on technique for our different events.

Jon was committed to each of us getting a personal best in every one of our meets. In the spring, we had seven meets against the seven other teams in our league. That meant I would have a chance to participate in the shot put and discus. There were still Saturday meets but I still didn't participate. My goal was to participate in a Saturday meet, and I always went for a personal best. This didn't mean placing first, second, or third. The point was to do my best, to push the people on my team to do their best, and for our team to win our meets. All of that happened. My friends Andy, Stan, and Mick were the ones who placed first, second, or third. Stan and Andy usually participated in the Saturday meets, along with my friend Mick. I finished last in nearly every one of the meets, but I didn't care because I always threw a personal best at shot put and discus, beating my own previous record.

At one of our meets, I was really angry with my head coach. It was a rainy day and he decided to allow only the top three people to participate. I wasn't among them. After the meet, I let the coach know how I felt.

I was shocked when one of the assistant coaches who coached me during indoor track started yelling at me, saying, "Bill, you are out of line! You had opportunities to participate in our Saturday events in the winter and you didn't take advantage of them. If you want to participate, be in the top three!" I spoke to Andy and Stan about it and they told me to let it go, so I did.

Our last meet of the year was against our rival, Upper Dublin. They were very good. The best on our team were competing, including my friends who did the shot put, discus and javelin. Stan told me he was going to win all three events, and he did. I had my best throws of the season by over a foot. In a practice throw of the discus, I had thrown it over one hundred feet. Unfortunately, I wasn't able to duplicate that kind of throw when the meet began. We ended up winning the track meet by less than ten points. That was the last time I would ever participate in a track meet. It was the only meet of the year that I didn't finish last. I was happy with my performance and proud of what I had accomplished over the two years I had participated in track. I had also lost over fifty-five pounds and ten inches off my waist. I had the respect and admiration of my teammates, classmates and teachers, and that felt very good.

The only meet left was our league championship. I didn't qualify but, luckily, many of my friends and teammates did. Our team ended up winning our league by over a hundred points, which was a lot. The girls' team also won their league, although it was a much closer contest for them. I believe they won by less than ten points. It was great to be able to celebrate with the girls after the meet was over. There were a lot of laughs and hugs. The week after our league championship was the district championship. I went to support my friends,

Stan and Andy. Neither of them met the qualifications for the state meet, but it was fun to hang out with them.

A few weeks after track season ended, the spring sports awards ceremony was held. It brought all the sports teams together—boys and girls. After each team announced their respective awards, the teams split up and had their own awards ceremonies. The coaches announced the best track athlete and the best field athlete. My friend Stan won best field athlete. Then the coaches had another award to give out. This was the coaches' award for dedication and perseverance. My coaches said some really great things about the person receiving this award. Then the head coach said, "The coaches' award for dedication and perseverance goes to Bill Deering."

I couldn't believe it. By this time, the girls' team was in the room along with all of my teammates, and everyone gave me a standing ovation. I walked up to the stage and stood before them with the award in my hand. This moment was so different from all the times I had stood out for stuttering; when I had heard only laughter and taunts. My new friends and teammates were now standing up, applauding, and cheering. Afterword, I thanked everyone and there were a lot of hugs. I still have that award. It always takes me back to that moment and how much it meant to me. I remember the two words on that award that I have come to know well in my life: dedication and perseverance.

The week before track season ended was senior prom, but I didn't go because, even with my testosterone shots, I had still never asked a girl out on a date. There were girls I wanted to ask, I just wasn't willing to face my fears. I also didn't have the money for a tuxedo because I didn't have a job like most of my friends did. I wasn't going to ask my mom because she was struggling just to get by. I didn't have my driver's license, either. Andy and Derek got on me the most about that, but not in a bad way. They asked me if I wanted one. I answered, "I guess I do but I'm afraid of driving and going on the highways, so I guess I'm not really that interested in getting my license."

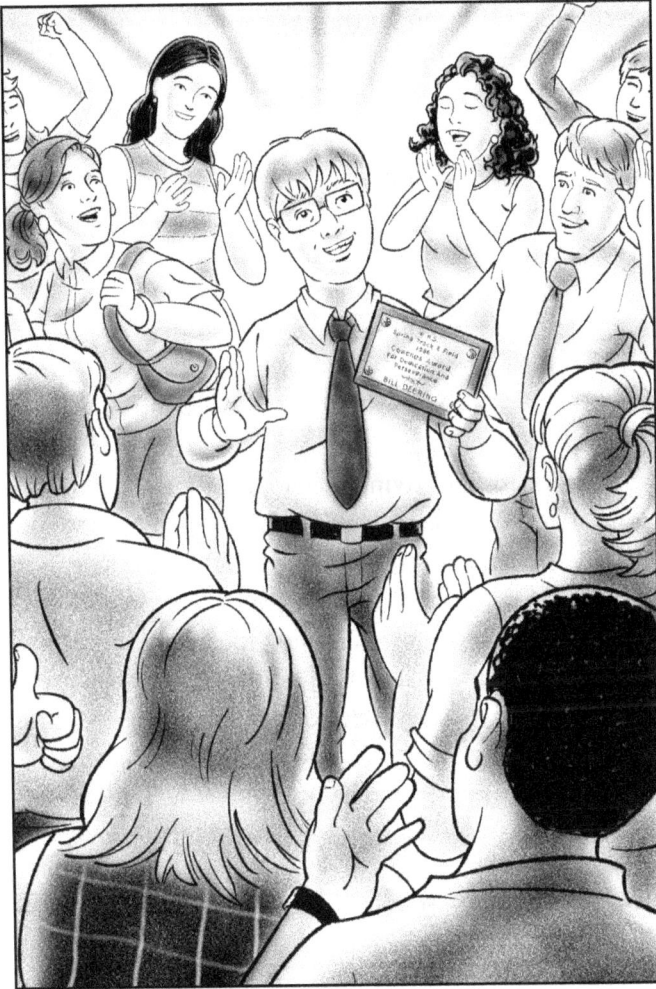

It was embarrassing, but I figured it really didn't matter. I wasn't going to my prom either way. While my friends were at the junior and senior prom, I was at home watching television. My friends told me all about it when I returned to school, and I wished I had been there with them.

By the time track season was over and the spring sports awards ceremony had taken place, I only had about one week of high school left. I couldn't believe the progress I had made in just two years. I mean, at the end of my sophomore year, my life looked hopeless. I had no friends, I was overweight, I was teased and bullied all the time, I had poor grades, I had family problems, and I stuttered very severely. And in just two years, my life changed drastically.

When I really looked at what made the difference, there were two things in particular: teamwork and perseverance. The first two years, I did everything by myself and wasn't involved in anything. I also wasn't really trying to improve my grades or be in good shape. The result was misery, depression, and isolation. The last two years, I took risks by getting involved in sports, stepping beyond my fear of stuttering, opening myself up to being loved and loving others, having fun, and learning to laugh at myself. I also worked hard to keep my commitments of improving my grades and getting myself in better shape. My self-confidence and self-esteem improved dramatically, and people really loved having me around.

My last week of high school was magical. I had received a letter in the mail a few weeks before about attending an awards program for student academics. I thought for sure they had the wrong person because my grades were definitely not honor society material. But I went anyway. My mom had to work late that night, so my friend Tony picked me up. I sat with him and some of the other people I knew from my class.

I watched as several of my classmates in the honor society received scholarship money and academic awards. Some of them got several. The program was almost over when my friend Fred said, "Big Bill, your name hasn't been called."

I looked at him and said, "I don't know what I'm doing here. There must be some reason why they invited me."

Sure enough, the last award of the night was for three students who showed the most improvement in the school, and I was one of them. Again, I was stunned. My friends and class-mates again applauded raucously for me, gave me high fives, and shook my hand. I got hugs from the girls in my class. That was my favorite part because attention from girls was so rare for me. I looked at the award and was really grateful and honored to have been picked. My mom had also arrived in time to see me receive it. She was very proud of me. That made two awards in two days: one for track and one for academics. I was on top of the world.

I thought about how far I had come from that kid who sat and cried in his room, or later when food was my only friend. Having something to finally be proud of was no small thing.

15

Moving On

My graduation date was June 11, 1986. I couldn't believe the day had actually arrived. I spent the previous two mornings going through graduation practice. All I could think about was graduating and seeing my friends. My friend Derek picked me up. I had gotten to know Derek from being on the football team and seeing him around school. We got to the cafeteria, where everyone was putting on their caps and gowns and giving each other hugs. I got to see several of my friends before we had to get in alphabetical order to enter the circular gym. Unfortunately, the air conditioning was broken in the gym. At ninety-plus degrees, the temperature outside was no better, even at 7:00 p.m. I gave up the idea of being cool and accepted that I was going to sweat a lot along with everyone else.

We entered the gym without anyone tripping and found our respective seats. Our principal made a few jokes about the oppressive heat, and then a few people spoke, including our valedictorian. My friend Annabelle sang one of the songs. Toward the end of the ceremony, a long list of scholarships were read out and awarded. Many of my classmates got several of them for their academic achievements. I was surprised for a third time when my name was called for one of them. I received a scholarship of two hundred and fifty dollars for being a good citizen, for being industrious, and for never giving up.

After all of the scholarships were given out, it was time to get our diplomas. The first row of students got up and the principal called each name one by one. Each of my classmates was handed a diploma and received rousing applause, some more than others. I knew I was supposed to be excited, but as the time drew closer and closer, I found myself getting very nervous. My heart was racing and I just wanted to get it over with. They called up the row ahead of me. I knew my row was next. Then students in my row started getting the call. There were maybe ten people ahead of me on my side and then another ten people on the other side. My friend Chase noticed me getting anxious and whispered to me, "Relax and enjoy the moment."

Before I knew it, I was next to go up on stage and our principal, Mr. Waterson, called my name.

"William Joseph Deering."

I walked across the stage to get my diploma and my classmates clapped very loudly for me. That calmed me down a bit and also gave me confidence. I raised my fists over my head like I was Rocky Balboa, and my classmates loved it. I made sure to enjoy the moment as Chase had suggested. I graduated with two hundred and seventy people that evening. After a while, no one cared about how hot and sweaty they were. When the last person walked off the stage with a diploma in hand, the principal announced, "Here is your Wissahickon class of 1986!"

With that, many classmates threw their caps in the air and began congratulating each other. As my classmates started leaving, I saw Guy Doyleson and gave him a hug, thanking him for all the encouragement and the coaching and for being my teacher. He was very proud of me. I walked up the steps, out of the gym, and into the lobby, where I found many of my classmates crying or embracing each other. I was moved by the realization of how much people meant to each other and needed each other. I was pleasantly surprised to receive so many handshakes from my male friends and so many hugs from my female friends. My friend Andy was a hugger, though. He hugged me instead of thumping me on the back or shaking hands like the others guys did. I didn't mind.

I walked out of the lobby and ran into my childhood friend Peter, who told me my parents and brothers were outside waiting for me. Making my way out of the hallway, I passed my friend Nina and gave her a hug. Next I saw Coach Hubbard. He embraced me, looked in my eyes and said, "Billy, I am very proud of you and how far you have come. I love you."

At that, I cried a little. His words had touched me, and I also knew I wouldn't see him every day anymore. I knew I would see Coach Hubbard sometime in the future, but it would be as an alumnus of the school. I was so happy and grateful that he was a part of my life. He made such a huge difference for me.

I was almost out of the hall when another friend, Lucy, approached and gave me a hug that lasted for over a minute. As I stood there, I had time to realize how much she and my other classmates had inspired me. I also thought for the first time that maybe I had inspired them too. If I had not pushed myself beyond my limitations, I never would have gotten to know them all. They would have remembered me only as that stuttering kid who never talked to anyone and got very fat. Instead, I was the kid who stuttered but got up there and talked anyway. I was the kid who gained fifty pounds to distract myself from my own misery but lost every bit of it through sheer determination. I was the kid who had difficulty in sports, but got in there and competed anyway. And I was the kid who appreciated every kindness they showed me and let them know it.

Finally, I exited the school and saw my parents and brothers. It was the first time I had shaken my dad's hand in a long time. I had blocked him out of my life for the last three years of high school. He said, "Bill, I am proud of you." Sadly, it meant a lot more coming from Coach Hubbard, who had become like a father to me. It was difficult, but I was gracious to my dad.

As in every high school, we had a tradition of writing in each other's yearbooks. Up until my senior year, I had never bought one. There didn't seem to be a point. But this year, my friends eagerly asked me if they could sign it. It was great to read what all my friends wrote to me. Coach Hubbard and Doc Doyleson also wrote great and inspiring comments. It was very fulfilling to read their words in particular because I had a lot of respect and admiration for them.

That night, I went to a party with my friend Derek and ran into a lot of people who had just graduated with me. I was also invited to a couple of pool parties my classmates were having. I was nervous about going to a pool party because I had never learned to swim. I went anyway and had fun at them regardless. No one seemed to mind. My friends were happy to have me there.

I spent a few days at the shore for senior week. I had my first taste of alcohol and it became clear immediately that I couldn't handle it. I got a bit out of hand one night and ended up making a fool of myself. The next day I got up and caught a bus to my house. I had quite a headache, but I was glad to be home. I wasn't sure when I would see my friends from high school again because many of them were headed to college after the summer. It was time for me to begin the next chapter of my life.

16

Starting Over

Even though I had improved my grades greatly the last two years of high school, they weren't high enough to get me into a four-year university. Instead, I spent the next two years at Montgomery County Community College.

I missed my high school friends terribly during the summer before my first semester of community college began. I especially missed my female friends and their great hugs. Because I never had the courage to ask any of them out on a date, I didn't have any of their phone numbers. I continued to run and would often go out of my way past my old high school, hoping I might see some of my friends from the football team. That happened occasionally but not as often as I would have liked. Sometimes during my runs I would see other people who had graduated with me, but instead of stopping they would honk their horns. Not being able to see my friends any longer was difficult for me. I missed them and didn't want to let go. I didn't want to move forward. I just wanted to go back to high school.

The summer ended and my friends were at their respective colleges and universities making new friends. It was time for me to begin my own college career at Montgomery County

Community College. I was very scared and nervous my first day because I didn't know anyone in my classes. I took four classes my first semester: accounting, statistics, history, and writing. I was worried that people were going to laugh at my stutter again, so I made sure not to say much. When I did speak, I would pick my words very carefully. All of my classes were extremely difficult for me, and they moved at a much faster pace in college. After the first day, I went to buy my books, and then I went to the library where I ran into a couple of friends from my high school, Tim and Adam. They had both graduated the year before me, but it was good to see people I knew.

In the summer of 1986, I decided to take a remedial writing class at Montco. I knew if I could get a grade of C or higher, I would be able to take the normal writing class. I had never really learned how to write in high school. I was always in remedial English classes and rarely had to write a paper or do research. Even though the writing class at my community college was remedial, I struggled mightily. I wasn't used to writing. I was frequently required to hand in two-page papers but just writing a sentence was a struggle for me, let alone an entire paragraph. I really hated it but I stuck with it. There was a tutoring center at the college even in the summer, so I got the help I needed. By the end of the six-week class, I received a C. I was so excited. It got me thinking that maybe I could handle college-level work.

That is not to say I didn't have doubts. I did. My parents said college would be a struggle for me. They were comparing me to my older brother, Jonathan, who was now a senior at the University of Pennsylvania. At the time, Penn was one of the premier universities in the country. He was walking those hallowed halls and I was in community college. But I wasn't going to let my parents dictate the level of success I achieved there.

About a month into the semester, I received a visit from a

state organization called the Office of Vocational Rehabilitation. I was not familiar with it. My mom had reached out to them to see if they would pay for speech therapy because I had expressed an interest in returning to therapy to overcome my stutter. A representative from this organization came to my mom's house. In addition to speech therapy, she said if I were able to maintain a C average, the organization would pay my entire tuition. It was a goal to shoot for. She also suggested that I switch from community college to business school due to my stutter and learning challenges, but I was committed to graduating from college.

The Office of Vocational Rehabilitation moved very slowly, which was frustrating because I wanted to start speech therapy right away. I still hadn't given up on overcoming my stutter, even though the hormone therapy was having no effect on it. Our application wasn't approved until late November. Even with the wait, however, this was a big deal for my mom and me because we couldn't afford therapy. Now this wonderful organization would pay for it until I overcame my stutter or until I felt comfortable at my level of fluency. It seemed like a great deal. I knew my mom was happy about it, and I was happy she didn't have to pay for my speech therapy or college tuition—as long as I kept a C average.

Speech therapy started in December of 1986 at a hospital in Norristown. I had to take two buses to get there, over ninety minutes each way. My therapist was a woman named Mrs. Crane. She shared with me that she had dabbled in math prior to becoming a speech therapist because she was good with numbers, but she gave it up because it wasn't satisfying to her. She wanted to help people struggling with speech disorders. I was happy to hear that.

I was very nervous during my first session because I hadn't had speech therapy since the ninth grade. I stopped after the first semester of my freshman year because it just wasn't helping. In fact, going to therapy seemed to make my speech worse. This was the first time in four years that I was willing to give it another chance. I was skeptical but decided to let go of past failures and do whatever it took to overcome my stutter. I still thought that if I didn't stutter, people would like me right away without my struggling to win them over. I could have a girlfriend. I could have self-confidence. My grades would be good enough to get into a four-year university. I had all that at stake in my therapy sessions. No pressure at all.

During my first session with Mrs. Crane, I stuttered so much, I could barely speak. How much I stuttered determined how badly I felt. If I didn't stutter much, I was more confident. If I stuttered a lot, my self-esteem and self-confidence were low. I had made such strides in high school to increase both, but it felt like I was starting over again.

After my first session, my therapist said, "Bill, I have an assignment for you. Read out loud for thirty minutes every night. This will help you slow down your speech and start to give you more confidence to speak."

I left that day and waited for the bus from Norristown back to Montgomery County Community College, where I would pick up my transfer bus to get myself home. I got home and shared with my mom that the therapist told me to read aloud every night for thirty minutes. Of course, I did it. I was willing to try anything. I started off with thirty minutes of reading aloud, but I increased it to an hour and, eventually, ninety minutes every night. I didn't care. I was willing to do whatever it took to get some relief from stuttering.

While I was going to speech therapy and attending community college, I was still in touch with Coach Hubbard. I shared with him that I was going to give my dad another chance. He thought that was a good idea. Even though I wasn't at Wissahickon any longer, I would still run new ideas past him nearly every time. I appreciated his opinion. My dad and I hadn't talked since my sophomore year other than a few brief exchanges. I had ignored him as much as possible. Coach

Hubbard became my father figure during the last two years of high school.

A few years earlier, I didn't think I would be able to talk to my dad again until he had apologized to my mom, and to me, for all the times he let us down. He never did apologize, but I was still willing to let him be a part of my life.

My dad was surprised when I agreed to go with him and my younger brother to watch my older brother, Jonathan, play at Franklin Field. Unfortunately, he didn't get a chance to play much because he was behind two all-American running backs. He didn't seem to mind, though. He enjoyed being part of a winning program. He could have started for any of the other Ivy League schools but decided on Penn instead. It seemed to be a good choice for him.

We started out slow. I saw my grandmother (my dad's mom) for the first time in three years. She was thrilled to see me, as were my aunt and my Uncle Bob. At first, it felt a little weird being around them and my dad at the same time, but I got over it. I didn't see my dad much, but it was a start. I think both of my brothers were happy to see that I was at least willing to give him another shot. My silent demeanor when he was around or when his name was mentioned had been the elephant in the room for long enough.

17

University of My Choice

As always, my main focus during my freshman year at community college was to overcome my stutter. I wanted to do well in my classes, too, but I wasn't very motivated to do so because I was spending so much time reading aloud so I could speak more fluently. My therapy was zipping along. I was listening to my therapist. I talked more slowly. I did whatever she suggested. Even though I had already proven to myself—or more correctly, the good friends and teachers I had in high school had proven to me—that I could be loved and admired despite my stutter, I kept thinking if I could just overcome it completely, once and for all, my life would be so much better. People would like me more. People would admire me. I would be loved. I would be appreciated. I would be able to start dating. People wouldn't laugh at me any longer. Girls would find me attractive and want to be around me. My self-esteem and self-confidence would improve dramatically. I would be proud of myself and many other people would be proud of me, too. I would have more friends. I didn't want to let anyone down. I had to keep pushing myself. I had to keep going. I had to keep my head up. I had so much riding on overcoming my stutter.

It was nearly the end of April and I was noticing quite a change in my fluency, as were my mom, dad, and brothers. Mrs. Crane was really working with me. It was time to start dealing with the situations that gave me the most trouble. I had avoided those situations for as long as I could remember. They included answering the phone, talking on the phone, introducing myself, ordering food in a restaurant, asking a stranger a question, and talking in front of groups of people. Having to face these fears was the most challenging part of speech therapy. I started with the first two. I began calling my friends from the track team who were now seniors in high school. I told them what I was doing, and they were happy to help.

I was still reading aloud for ninety minutes every day. Now I was spending two to three hours per week speaking to friends on the phone, too. It wasn't easy but I did it. Additionally, I practiced picking up the phone and saying "hello" fifty to one hundred times every day. When I first started answering the phone, my mom and younger brother were surprised. But I was determined to be able to say hello without stuttering. Sure enough, after a month I was able to answer the phone fluently nearly every time. I was moving right along. I just kept gathering my courage and tackling my challenges head-on.

By far the most difficult challenge was ordering food in a restaurant. I dreaded it above everything else. Growing up, I had never ordered for myself. My parents, brothers, or friends would always order for me. Now I was ready to take on this challenge. Every time I met with my therapist, we went to the hospital cafeteria and I ordered tea. No matter how much I practiced and rehearsed to myself saying, "I will take some tea, please," I just couldn't say the words without stuttering. And then it happened. One day, after several sessions, I was able to say, "I will take tea," without stuttering. I was so happy anyone watching would have thought that I had just won the lottery. I could have floated home. I couldn't wait to tell my mom the good news.

The more I practiced, the more fluent I became. My self-confidence improved dramatically. After seven and a half months, my therapist told me I had overcome my stutter and was being discharged. It was a joyous day for me: July 29, 1987. My therapist reminded me that I still had to practice all of my problem situations consistently, and that if I did, my fluency would continue.

By now, school was over. I had finished my first year of community college with a 1.75 grade-point average, which meant that I earned three C's and a D each semester. On one hand, I was consistent, but on the other, my grades fell short of what I needed to achieve my goal: going to the four-year university of my choice. I didn't want to go to just any university. In the summer of 1987, I started looking at my goals. What did I really want to achieve? I thought to myself, "I want to get a B average because I have never gotten a B average before in my life." I wanted to keep expanding and do something I had never done before.

Over the summer of 1987, I ran into an old high school friend who said, "Bill, I think it's great that you overcame your stutter, but you are still going to have to work hard. There is no way to get around working hard." He was right. I applied the same attitude to my grades that I had to my stutter. I was willing to do whatever it took for me to get my grades where they needed to be.

I also planned to do everything I had done in high school. I could study every day and talk to my professors after class, but I knew to be successful I was going to have to talk to the people in my classes. That meant I was going to have to risk stuttering and being laughed at. But I had already been down this road and not only survived but thrived, so I was willing to take on the challenge. Besides, I had just overcome a very severe stutter and felt like I was on cloud nine. Nothing could stop me.

When I came back for my second year at community

college, I was feeling very confident because I had my stutter under control and I had a plan. I was taking five classes per semester. I studied every day. I was prepared for my exams. I talked to people in my classes. I asked for help when I needed it. I was willing to take the risk of stuttering and feeling embarrassment and humiliation for the opportunity to make new friends and feel comfortable around other people. It paid off.

My classmates in science were interested in knowing me regardless of whether I stuttered or not. They thought it was great that I had gone to speech therapy, but for them it didn't matter how much or how little I stuttered. That was such a relief for me. Not all of my classes were like that, though. I still felt like I had to keep my guard up because I was never sure when someone might think my stutter was funny. I was always on the lookout for that possibility. I met people in my second year of college who laughed at me. I thought they had either never heard anyone stutter before or they were just ignorant. Either way, it didn't matter to me because I was on a mission to get a B average. I worked and studied harder than ever.

That semester I didn't reach a B average. I fell just short with a 2.86 grade-point average. Even though that was the best GPA I had ever earned, in high school or college, and was a full point higher than my GPA from the year before, I wasn't satisfied. I knew I could do better. I was determined to break a B average in the upcoming spring semester. My overall GPA was over 2.0, which was all I needed to get into a four-year university, but my goal was to go to the university of my choice and not settle for less.

In my spring semester, I had five classes again. They were all challenging. One of them was music education. I thought for sure it was going to be my easiest class. I was wrong. It ended up being the hardest. My professor in music liked to give essay tests, which wasn't good for me because I struggled when taking notes. My listening and note-taking skills didn't seem to be up to par with the rest of my class. On my first exam I got a C-minus, which wasn't what I wanted. One of my classmates who had been sitting next to me received an A. I ran into that classmate later in the library. I approached and asked if I could sit with him and he said yes. He told me he was having difficulty with learning math. I responded, "I will help you learn math if I can borrow your notes for music class." He said that was a great idea. With my help, he achieved A's and B's in math and I got solid B's in music.

It was during that same year that he took me and my brothers out to dinner at a seafood restaurant and introduced us to his fiancé. Lisa was less than five feet tall and she seemed very nice. The thing that struck me most about her was how easy it was to speak with her. My father noticed that I wasn't stuttering anymore and said he was happy for me. It was still hard for me to forget how he had yelled at me to "spit it out already," instead of helping me, but I thanked him anyway.

Lisa married my dad the next year. They lived in New Jersey. I met my stepsister, Julie, and stepbrother, Ted. They were twelve and fourteen at the time. I didn't really spend much time with them until they were older. I saw Lisa and my dad very infrequently through my college years. It wasn't a hard adjustment to make because I had grown accustomed to not seeing him during the years when I avoided talking to him.

At the end of that second year of community college, my classmate graduated with his associate degree. I received a 3.14 GPA the second semester and achieved my goal of a B average. I also got accepted into the four-year university of my choice. I went to West Chester University in Pennsylvania. My mom was proud of what I had accomplished, but I was prouder. I thought about the friend from high school who told me there's no way around hard work, even without a stutter. He was right. That philosophy helped me persevere during those long nights of studying when I would have preferred to be doing anything else at all.

I still had my stutter under control, but it had gotten a

little worse because I wasn't practicing all the situations my therapist had recommended. I was so focused on getting better grades that I became complacent with the fluency strategies that had gotten me to where I was at that time.

Over the summer, I worked at 7-Eleven. It was close to where I lived so I could walk there. Occasionally, I had to work in another store three miles away and would jog there and jog back home. The summer went by very quickly. Before I knew it, I was about to embark on a new adventure—attending West Chester University. I was unable to find housing on campus, so I lived in a rooming house. I was nervous because it was my first time on my own, and even though there were a few people I knew, I didn't know when I would see them. Basically, I was alone, which made me scared and anxious. I didn't have my own car, so my mom graciously drove me with all of my stuff to the place I was going to live for the next year.

When I arrived, my roommate was already there. He and I had spoken on the phone prior to meeting in person and I had already explained that I stuttered, but I had forgotten to tell him my name during that conversation. He shook my hand and introduced himself to my mother and me as Alvin. I said, "I am B-b-b-b-b-b-b-b-b-b-b-b-b-b-b-b-b-b-b-b-b-b-b-b-b-b-b-b-b-b-b-b-b-b-b-b-b-bi-i—i-i-i-i-i-i-i-i-i-i-i-i-i-i-i-i-i-i-i-i-i-i-l-l-l-l-l-l-l-l-l-l-l-l-l-l-l-l." Finally, after what seemed like an eternity to me, I said, "My name is Bill." Alvin didn't flinch.

He said, "Nice to meet you, Bill," and offered to help my mom and me get all of my stuff into the room. When we were done, I walked my mom out and gave her a hug. I was sad at first and felt lonely because my mom wasn't there with me. I was used to being home with her. That first day, I met several of my housemates. I tried my best not to stutter too much. They were friendly but I was very apprehensive about being around so many people I didn't know. I wanted to find a place where I could be left alone but there was nowhere to go, so I just kept trying to go with the flow.

I went with Alvin and some of my other housemates to a welcome picnic for incoming freshmen and transfers. While my housemates talked amongst themselves and looked at the young women, I tried my best to be invisible. I stopped talking altogether and ate my food. After the picnic, as I headed home with them, some decided to go to a dance and invited me. I walked over with them, but when it was time to go inside, I decided I didn't want to and walked back to my room. I thought to myself, "Maybe it's a mistake for me to be here." I really missed being at home with my mom and my younger brother. I was safe there. I was disappointed with myself that after all the strides I had made academically and socially, and after gaining so much control over my stutter, I still sometimes felt like that kid who was afraid of being laughed at and humiliated. The bully—my own fear—had found me again. I thought, "Would I ever escape? I had proven to myself over and over that I was likable and that people could be kind to me even with my stutter. These people were no different. Why was I afraid and nervous again?" I decided it had to get better. After all, the alternative—quitting the university, going back home, and living my life in hiding—was far worse than facing my fears.

Classes began the next day. I walked into West Chester as a math major. I didn't take it easy my first semester; I took five hard classes—linear algebra, calculus, introduction to computer science, French, and economics—sixteen credits total. I don't know what I was thinking. My roommate, Al, had four classes and only one of his classes was challenging for him. Of course, with that many classes, nobody could ever argue if I needed time to study when they asked me to go to a dance or a party. It was a great excuse to avoid social events.

Fortunately, after the first few weeks, I got a lot more comfortable with my housemates and began to talk with them.

There were eighteen people in my house—three women and fifteen guys. Their ages ranged from eighteen to twenty-three years old. There were nine rooms with two people to a room and two bathrooms. All of my housemates liked to party and drink beer. That seemed to be the common ground for them. Al loved to drink. He liked getting drunk three or four days per week. I wasn't much into partying in high school and hadn't really done much drinking, except for that night at the shore when I made a fool of myself.

I got along really well with one of the other guys in the house, Zeke. He was a crazy guy, but I seemed to connect most with him. I ate the majority of my meals with him and Alvin. If I missed a meal with one of my housemates, I would never go by myself. It was too frightening. I also didn't want anyone to think I didn't have any friends. What I did instead was go across the street where there was a Burger King, but I would never order the food I really wanted. I chose the food items that were easiest for me to say, even if it was food I didn't like, because I didn't want the people who worked there to laugh at my stutter. What I wanted to order was a burger. Instead I ordered French fries and a chef salad so I would have something in my stomach until I could go to the cafeteria with my friends the following day.

To say I struggled socially would be a severe understatement. The only time I felt comfortable enough to talk to anyone other than my housemates was either when we had a party at our house, or when I had a few drinks in me. I found that I was able to relax after a beer or two. I didn't stutter as much and if I did, it didn't seem to bother me as much. After these parties, I would feel hopeful that I had made a few new friends aside from my housemates, but most of the people I met didn't remember me when I would see them on campus.

If I wasn't with my housemates, at the cafeteria, or at our house, I was at the library studying. I dropped out of computer science because it was just too much to take in my first semester. I should have taken easier classes my first year. I figured my talent for arithmetic would help me in my math classes. I was wrong. My calculus professor was hard-nosed and didn't believe in giving anyone breaks. He said, "Calculus takes a lot of blood, guts, and hard work." A 60 was a D, a 70 was a C, an 80 was a B and anything above a 90 was an A. If you got a 59, you failed. No breaks. You did the work and either passed or failed. I studied hard but failed every exam. My professor put questions on exams that included other types of math such as geometry, algebra, and trigonometry. It was irrational, but I often felt like I was being tricked and had no real chance of passing his class.

I wasn't ready for linear algebra, either. The people in my class all seemed to live, breath, and eat math. I didn't hold math in that regard. I just wanted to get through it and move on to the next class. I should have dropped that one, too. It would have saved me a lot of aggravation and frustration. I never knew any of the answers when the teacher would ask the class questions. I got a 56 on my first exam. I followed that up with a 46. On my third exam I got a 10. Yep, 10 out of 100. I basically had to get a perfect score on my take-home exam and final just to get a D. I thought if my professor gave me the take-home exam before Thanksgiving, my friend Joe, who attended Johns Hopkins University, also as a math major, could do the exam for me. Joe was phenomenal at math. Unfortunately, my professor didn't give us the take-home exam until we returned from Thanksgiving break. I took one look at the test, ripped it into little pieces, and threw it in the trash. I was conceding to get an F in linear algebra. In fact, I stopped going to the class altogether. It was no surprise when I failed linear algebra as well as calculus.

I had a hard time understanding my economics professor's accent, and many of my classmates did, too. He was originally from Africa. All of his exams were multiple-choice. I thought that would make the exams easier. It didn't. I did manage to squeeze out a D in his class, though.

I said very little in my classes to hide my stutter. As in high school, though, I couldn't avoid participation in French class. I didn't know when I was going to be called upon so I was always on edge. I did the best I could. I struggled to be fluent and hide my stutter as much as possible. I received my highest first-semester grade in that class—a C.

Besides going to classes and hanging out with my house-mates, I did very little. However, I did something a little crazy my first semester at West Chester. My cousin was getting married in October of 1988 and he invited my entire family. My roommate Alvin suggested that I get a new haircut. At the time, my haircut was similar to Richie Cunningham's from the TV show *Happy Days*. I looked like a young, clean-cut guy. Alvin, who I had discovered had a crazy side, suggested that I get a flattop for my cousin's wedding. My mom picked me up on a Thursday night and drove me home. She told me I had to get a haircut. The next morning, I walked down to the barbershop and my friend's dad, Mr. Rotini, asked me how I wanted it cut.

"I want a flattop," I said.

Stunned, he asked, "Are you sure?"

"Yes, I'm sure," I replied, not entirely certain of what I was getting myself into.

Within five minutes, my haircut was done. I looked like a new recruit for the marines. I paid Mr. Rotini and walked home. My brothers laughed but my mom didn't find it funny at all. She told me I was going to stick out. I told her there's nothing wrong with sticking out. It turns out I was the only one at the wedding with a crew cut or flattop and I got a lot of compliments. Al told me if I got a flattop, more women would be attracted to me, so I listened. I was disappointed that no women threw themselves at me at my cousin's wedding. So much for that theory.

When I returned to school that Sunday night, my room-mate Alvin was shocked, and so was my friend Zeke. They and my other housemates couldn't believe I had gone through with it. I was a bit shocked myself. There I was, a formerly normal-looking, twenty-year-old guy looking like a marine going to boot camp.

On November 1, 1989, I turned twenty-one years old. I was now at the legal age to consume alcohol. The problem was I still didn't have a driver's license because I was still afraid to drive so I couldn't get into any bars. Having my license didn't seem like a big deal to me. Instead of going to a bar, I hung out with Alvin and my other housemates. I got a six-pack of Moosehead. Alvin, Zeke and I also bought Maddog 20/20 Orange Jubilee—a really cheap wine. It didn't take a lot to get me drunk. By 11:00 p.m., I was passed out in my bed. The next morning at 10:00 a.m., I had my linear algebra class. This was before I had stopped going. I woke up at around 9:30 a.m. Alvin was already awake and asked me where I was going.

"To my class," I responded.

"Go take a look in the mirror," he said.

I looked in the mirror and there were drawings of male genitals on both of my cheeks and the number 666 on my forehead. They had even decorated my legs with similar "art." I was upset at first, but then Alvin and I started laughing.

I knew this wasn't something I could wash off in a minute or perhaps even an hour, so I said, "I guess I'm not going to class." Getting the permanent marker off of my face and legs was not only a very lengthy process and painful process, but I had to admit it was kind of funny. Besides, if I stayed mad, I would have been the only one not laughing.

18

Communication Disorders

Not everything was hunky dory at the Cider abode, as our house was called. Alvin and I had our challenges. He kicked me out of the room a lot when women were over. That got old real quick. While I was bored hanging out in a hallway, he was having the time of his life. By the end of first semester, we were both in need of a vacation from each other. Over Christmas break, my parents expressed concern over my .7 grade-point average. They told me to get myself together. I could understand their frustration. The previous year I had gotten a B average and now I was facing a long, uphill battle with my grades. When I returned in January of 1989, I decided it would be better for me to take some easier classes and do a lot less partying. I took four classes. None of them were math.

Me not partying did not sit well with my housemates. They were used to me drinking and having fun with them. But I couldn't keep going down that road. My relationship with Mark, one of my housemates, started to turn a bit sour. A lot of his jokes were getting old. I discovered he had a nasty streak in him the time he told me I would never have a girlfriend. He said, "Bill, what woman would ever want to go out with you with that stutter?" That really hurt.

After he made that comment, I didn't want anything to do with him. In fact, I was so pissed off I wanted to punch him out. I started to spend more weekends at home with my mom and younger brother than at college. I just didn't want to be around Alvin and some of my other housemates. I was still stuttering very severely. I was still struggling in my classes. Even though I didn't have any math classes, I still had to work hard just to pass. I spent less and less time at the place where I lived, only going there to sleep.

As the semester came to a close, I counted down the days until I could go home. I had made a couple of friends in the house, but none outside our group. I did improve my grades. I received a 1.92 GPA, which was better than before but still far below what I had hoped to get. Alvin and I made the best of a bad situation and were amicable for the most part. However, he made sure to let me know that he received a 3.5 grade-point average and that he rarely studied. Nice, huh? But I learned something from Alvin. Some people are your best friend as long as you amuse them, but when you stop, their true natures comes out. Now I knew to look out for that in the future.

Alvin, Zeke, and a few other people from the house decided to get an apartment together. I was glad I wouldn't have to room with Alvin again. As angry as I was with him, I did miss the times when we got along and hoped we might become friends again somehow. I hadn't had many friends I could laugh with like that, so it hurt to see it end, no matter how bad his behavior was. Another part of me was glad to be moving on.

The summer of 1989 was uneventful for me except for an accidental meeting with my friend Andy Rotini. He and his brother were also at West Chester University with me. They had an apartment off-campus. During my entire first year, I only saw Andy once. He was with his girlfriend. That summer, I worked at the 7-Eleven close to my mom's house again to earn additional income to support myself at college. I still didn't have a car, a license, or any interest in getting either.

Over the summer, I received a letter in the mail from West Chester University. It wasn't a good one. The letter basically stated, *Bill Deering, you have a year to bring up your grade-point average to over a 2.0 or we will kick you out of school.* That was a bit of a shock for my mom and me. After the panic passed, though, I thought of it as an opportunity to bounce back and to show others and myself that I can really do college work. I decided in that moment that I was done with math and that I was going to find another major that really lit me up.

I decided to go into speech therapy. It was the obvious choice. I figured I could help a lot of people because of my own stuttering and familiarity with the subject. When it was time for me to pick my fall courses, I signed up for French, Educational Counseling, statistics, science, and Introduction to Communication Disorders. I had five classes for a total of fifteen credits. I figured out that to bring my current grade-point average from a 1.28 to a 2.0 in a year, I was going to have to generate a 2.7 for the 1989-1990 school year. Given the year I had just experienced, I had my work cut out for me. I went back to living at the Cider rooming house again. Luckily for me, my roommate was respectful and also into studying. He and I got along well. I decided I was going to study every day like I did when I was in community college.

My classes were challenging. My favorite was Introduction to Communication Disorders. It was a general class that gave an overview of all the things I would learn if I decided to major in that field. The one thing I enjoyed the most was being the only guy in the class. Male classmates were always more likely to laugh at me than girls were, so this was a relief for me. I didn't mind participating in that class.

My stutter had returned with a vengeance. I found out there was a speech clinic on campus I could go to for free, so I decided to give speech therapy another try. I thought maybe I could overcome my stutter again.

My therapist was a senior and an undergraduate therapist.

Her advisor happened to be the chairperson of the program. They worked with me more on how I felt about stuttering and less on techniques. This helped to a certain degree, but neither the therapist nor the advisor had ever stuttered. When they told me stuttering wasn't a big deal, they had no idea what they were talking about. But I listened as much as I could. It was good to be able to talk to someone again about stuttering.

When I wasn't at therapy or my classes, I spent time with my housemates. Thankfully, they weren't nearly as crazy as the ones from the year before. In the fall, I watched football games with them and we all went to the cafeteria together. That year, I didn't spend much time with Alvin and Zeke. I saw them on campus and hung out with them a little, but I knew at the end of the night, I could leave and go home to sleep. Other than that, I wasn't very sociable. I wasn't involved with any student organizations on campus. I went to my classes, studied, had lunch, studied again, had dinner, studied some more, and then slept. That was the routine day in and day out. I had no choice. I didn't want to get kicked out of school.

My hard work paid off. I received a 2.67 grade-point average in the fall. I had now raised my overall average to a 1.8. But I still had to continue to work hard in my classes. In the spring, I got a 2.73 and reached my goal of a C average. That meant I could stay in school. I brought my grades from a 1.28 to a 2.05 in one year. I was proud of myself and all the work I had put in to make that happen.

Even though I didn't have any friends outside of my rooming house, there was a woman in my French class I liked. Unfortunately, I never had the courage to tell her I liked her. She was three years younger than me and very friendly. As always, my thought process was that it was better to be safe and not take the chance of being turned down. I still think of her now and then, wondering if I might have become closer to her if I had just had the courage to ask her out and express my feelings.

By the time my second year at West Chester University had ended, I was officially a Communication Disorders major. I had also decided to get an apartment with my housemates, Albert and Doug. They were cousins. They had a friend named Howie who would be joining us as well. I was up for something new.

I was heading into my third year at West Chester University. When Howie and I first started out as roommates, we were very chummy but it didn't take long for our friendship to go south. We were complete opposites. Howie was loud and obnoxious. He said anything for a laugh regardless of how his joke was received by others. He also smoked and drank excessively. I drank occasionally but was quiet and kept to myself. It didn't take long to realize that I had made a mistake in my roommate choice. Howie and I eventually started arguing and the tension mounted daily. I could have chosen to make other arrangements but instead I made the best of a bad situation. I learned two lessons: 1. be certain to know someone well before getting into a yearlong lease with him, and 2. I should surround myself with people who are positive and supportive.

My classes were difficult that first semester. They were the classes that counted toward my major. I also had statistics, earth science, and English literature. The person who usually taught Voice Disorders was on sabbatical. Instead, my professor was Dr. Steers. He was renowned for his work with people who stuttered. He led the course like it was a graduate class. He held pop quizzes. He talked very fast and I didn't take good notes. I ended up failing that class.

My Anatomy and Physiology for Speech Mechanisms class was just as hard. My professor was funny and likable and told some really silly jokes. Everyone seemed to like him. I studied very hard for his classes. There was a lot to learn. I always studied for my tests by memorizing. That usually worked, but it didn't work in anatomy class. I failed every exam, including the final one. Five exams in a row. The thing that saved me was a term paper. Even with that grade, I still only managed a D, which meant I was going to have to repeat both Voice Disorders and the anatomy class the next fall.

One of the good things that came out of being in those classes was that I got to study with some women. I was the only guy in the major. Unfortunately, the study group didn't help me much with my classes.

My other courses were just as hard. Statistics was very confusing. My professor helped as much as he could but I still received a C. My earth science professor was also a mentor of mine and I thought his class was going to be easy, or that he would take it easy on me. Neither was the case. I had to work hard in that class.

Then there was English literature. I thought for sure that this class was going to be easy but it was one of the hardest classes I had ever taken. Breaking with tradition, I actually opened my mouth and made a new friend named Chas. Chas had long, blond hair and a beard. He was very focused on his grades. He spent many hours studying. I was impressed by his work ethic. He helped me with some homework in one of my classes. He reinforced the philosophy of working hard and persisting until I reached my goals. Out of the few people I had met that year, Chas was by far the nicest, most gracious, and helpful. He was very positive. He and I became friends and hung out. In May of 1991, he told me that he was graduating in the fall of that year. I was happy for him.

I didn't have a lot of friends in college. Besides Chas and my former housemates, Alvin and Zeke, I didn't hang out with too many other people. I was still staying in my comfort zone and getting by. My fear of asking a woman out and being laughed at was as strong as it had been when I was a sophomore in high school. Despite the strides I had made, I just couldn't get past it. It was easier to hide from the world than risk that kind of humiliation.

That year, I started spending more time with Alvin and

Zeke. Now that we weren't housemates anymore, Alvin and I seemed to get along much better. Zeke and I had always gotten along and it was good to see him. By now, he was in a serious relationship with Annie. Both of them were on track to graduate in May of 1992. I, on the other hand, was now looking at May of 1993. My most important lesson from my third year at West Chester was that I needed to stop doing things by myself. I had discovered in high school that being part of a team made a big difference. So far in college, the experience of having a team was definitely missing. I intended to change that.

Besides being in my classes, I was also going to speech therapy. My therapist was a graduate student who was studying for her master's degree, and her advisor was Dr. John Steers. He was the same Dr. Steers who was my professor of Voice Disorders the prior year. It was his class I had failed. As I spent time with my therapist and Dr. Steers, I discovered that Dr. Steers really did care about how I was doing. Although I struggled mightily with his teaching methods, he supported and encouraged me on a personal level. He told me about a device called the Fluency Master, which he said could significantly improve my speech. I was a bit skeptical, but I watched the videos he showed me. It was unbelievable to see the before and after videos of people who went through his program. I really wanted this device, but it was a total of fifteen hundred dollars. I wasn't interested in spending that much money on a device that *might* work for me. My speech was up and down. On my good days, I felt very confident and joyous, like I could accomplish anything. On my bad days, I felt defeated, sad, and lonely. I had been wishing for so long that my stuttering would just go away and never come back, I was tired of wishing and sometimes felt like I was stuck with it for life. Still, the seemingly magical Fluency Master kept returning to my thoughts.

19

Fluency Master

Entering my fourth year at West Chester I was very enthusi-
astic about repeating the two courses I needed to graduate.
I could finally see a path to graduation. I also had two other
classes. I was back to living at the Cider abode where I had
lived my first two years, except now I had my own room and
didn't have to deal with a roommate. I got along with my
housemates, too. None of them were too crazy. One of my
housemates, Roger, went on and on about a camp where he
had been a counselor for several years. It was called Golden
Slipper Camp. I listened to the same stories over and over again
but didn't mind. He was a great guy. He was very focused
on becoming a teacher and had a real passion for kids. With
my housemates, I felt safe. We hung out and went to meals
together.

All of my classes were very difficult again. I was happy to
discover that I was again the only guy in my speech therapy
classes. I had the same professor for anatomy class and a
different professor for Voice Disorders. One morning before
anatomy class, a woman introduced herself to me. Her name
was Shirley. She and I quickly became friends. She didn't care

that I stuttered. She was already in a serious relationship, but I didn't care. I was just happy to have a new friend.

About eight weeks into the semester, I dropped my other two classes and just focused on my two major classes. I had taken another anatomy exam and failed that one, too, even though I studied very hard for it. I just couldn't figure out how to pass the class. In fact, my anatomy teacher called me into his office and said, "Bill, I think you ought to find another major. I know you want to make it in this one, but you have failed six exams in a row. At least think about it."

I met with the department chairperson, who said, "Bill, you are really struggling in this major and this is undergraduate work. How are you going to make it through to get your master's degree and become a speech therapist? Is it really worth the struggle?" I said nothing. I went home and cried in my room. Sometimes I just got so tired of everything being so hard, I had to let myself cry it out. I spoke with my dad about it and he encouraged me to keep going. He told me I could do it. It felt good to have his support. All the messy and complicated emotions surrounding him were still there, but his encouragement seemed to be his way of trying to make amends. I hung up the phone, wiped the tears away, and got back to work.

I called my friend Chas, who suggested I start recording my classes; so that's what I started doing. I bought a mini tape recorder and taped my lectures. Then I went home and listened to the tapes over and over again until I could transcribe all the notes into my notebook. I also reached out to my professors and to the people in my classes and asked them for support. They were willing to help me as well, just like back in high school. Although I only had two classes, I was studying five to six hours per day. I even went to the library to borrow another anatomy book so I could follow along with my notes and look at the pictures in the book to understand the processes. I really wanted to make it to graduation and was willing do whatever it took to get there.

It was time for my next anatomy exam. By now, my professor allowed me to take my exams untimed. I took the exam and received a 73. After failing six exams in a row, it felt good to receive that score. I had finally passed an exam, which gave me the confidence that I could do the work. I did a little better on each one after that. My final exam was multiple-choice and I studied my butt off for that one. I got an 85 and a C-plus in the class. I was very proud of myself. I also squeezed out a C in my Voice Disorders class.

Outside of my classes, I still didn't really do much except hang out with my housemates. I didn't have an interest in joining any clubs for fear that it would take too much time away from my studies. Sometimes I hung out with Zeke and Alvin, who had both become good friends again by now.

The following semester, I had two more classes: Language Disorders and Clinical Principles. I was still attending speech therapy at the clinic on campus. Dr. Steers was now the advisor to the graduating students. I was glad to have him. He was always willing to speak with me. The master's degree student was a woman. She was great. When I began to struggle in my classes, she suggested that I get tutoring, so that's what I did.

I had to study a lot longer than my classmates. Everything seemed to be much harder for me than for others. Clinical Principles was hard because I had to create age-appropriate activities for potential clients that I would be seeing in my final year. I wasn't very creative and had no idea what to do. I really struggled with that project. Luckily, it wasn't my entire grade. I always managed to do well on my exams. I was fortunate to have great tutors who would make recommendations or offer simple ideas I could use.

My other class was Language Disorders. The professor I had for that class was very dynamic and an expert in that field. Even though I was able to tape her classes and rewrite all of my notes, her exams were very challenging. Additionally, I had to do research and write a paper. She let me pick the topic, which was nice of her. It was only the third or fourth paper I had been assigned in my college career.

During that semester, I received a call from my dad, who said he would pay for me to get the Fluency Master and go through Dr. Steers' program in March of 1992. He had finally accepted that I had a real problem I couldn't control. He knew I still hadn't forgiven him for what he did, but offering his support, morally and financially, was his way of trying to fix things. I accepted his gift and thanked him.

It was a Sunday in mid-March when I finally had the opportunity to go through the Fluency Master program. I had to walk almost three miles to get to the location, but I didn't care. It was a beautiful, sunny day and there was hope at the end of this road. There was a part of me that didn't think the Fluency Master would work for me, but I ignored it and kept walking. The program itself was five hours. When I got to the West Chester location, there were three other people who stuttered that were going through the program as well. It was one of the few times that I met other people who stuttered. For most of my life, I actually thought I was the only one, and that it was a very rare condition. It isn't. About one percent of people in the world stutter, and that's a lot of people.

Dr. Steers led the program along with some other master's degree candidates who wanted experience with the Fluency Master. From the moment I put on the Fluency Master until I took it off five hours later, I couldn't believe how much more fluently I was able to say my words. It was amazing. My stutter was gone. I left that March afternoon feeling more hopeful than I had ever been before that someday I would be free of stuttering. It was like my fluency challenges had been resolved. I had to wait two weeks to receive my own Fluency Master. Those two weeks could not go by quickly enough. When I finally got it, my classmates noticed a difference immediately.

They made comments like, "Bill, your speech sounds so clear and you're not stuttering!" Those comments felt so good. In my heart, I was jumping for joy and giving myself high-fives. I couldn't believe how great I felt. Even when I did stutter, it didn't bother me too much. I just wanted that high to last for the rest of my life.

While celebrating this victory, I still had to deal with how difficult my classes were. It took a lot of time to prepare for exams, write my paper for Language Disorders, and prepare my clinical notebook for future opportunities as a speech therapist. I was still getting tutored. I was still going to therapy except now the focus was on the language challenges I had. I was happy with my progress and had a great camaraderie with my all-female classmates. They were some of my biggest supporters, especially my friend Shirley. She lived right down the street from me and we walked to class together. She encouraged and believed in me. That meant a lot. I ended up getting a B in Clinical Principles and a C-plus in Language Disorders. I was pleased with my progress. Many of my professors were very impressed with my efforts. They admired my courage and perseverance.

My dad was much more supportive of me in my college years at Montgomery County Community College and West Chester University. He showed his loved to me in many ways. He wasn't one to say "I love you" but showed his love through his actions. We had lunch a few times a year during my time at West Chester. He paid for my tuition and housing at West Chester for a few years. After so much bad blood between us, I appreciated him making the effort to be supportive and encouraging in my college years. I had changed for the better and he had, too.

In the summer of 1992, with the support of my housemate Roger, I signed on to work at the Golden Slipper Camp in Stroudsburg, Pennsylvania, that he talked so much about. I was going to be way outside of my comfort zone. I was hired to be a camp counselor for eight weeks. I still didn't have a car so my mom drove me up to the camp five days before the campers were to arrive. I didn't meet my co-counselor until my first day of training. His name was Tim Michaels and he was from Midland, Texas. He had just graduated high school. He was a pretty mellow guy. He was average in height but about one hundred and seventy pounds of solid muscle. We got along really well from the moment we met.

I brought my Fluency Master and felt pretty comfortable being at the camp. However, a few days before the campers got there, the battery in my device went dead and there was no place close enough to get it replaced. When that happened, I realized how much emphasis I had been putting on being fluent. I immediately became very scared and nervous again. I not only had to deal with potentially stuttering severely but also the possibility of the kids at this camp laughing at me. Tim was great, though. He kept assuring me everything would work out. We had a group of ten eight-year-olds. When we got the kids back to the bunk and introduced ourselves, I let everyone know that I stuttered and would appreciate them not laughing at me. They all agreed to be respectful. That was such a relief.

It dawned on me that I should have said the same thing to my classmates on the first day of school all those years ago when I was growing up. It might have had the same effect. Talking about my stuttering would have worked much better than trying to wish it away and worrying about what everyone else was thinking.

On the first night, all the counselors had to introduce themselves. Even though I just had to say two words—Uncle Bill—I was very nervous. I wanted to say my name without stuttering, which was always a great victory for me. I was relieved when I did say my name fluently. I discovered that most of the kids I met that summer didn't care that I stuttered, nor did my fellow counselors. I was still the person who had the most difficulty with it and didn't have a solution for accepting it in myself.

Even though I struggled with my stutter that summer, I persevered. I participated in all the activities. I assisted other counselors. I had fun. I made new friends. One of my new friends was a camper. Her name was Holly and she was four-teen years old. Every time I saw her, she would ask for a "hello hug" and I would oblige. After camp, we stayed in touch by writing to each other.

I confided the most in my friend and co-counselor, Tim. In just eight short weeks, we had become good friends. We stayed in touch, too. I learned over the summer that I could be friends with people regardless of our age difference.

I was excited to get back to West Chester University for my final year of college. I needed just five classes to graduate, but that was going to take a year because one of my major classes was only offered in the spring. I still felt like I had a lot to prove to myself and to some of the professors in my major. I took two classes the first semester. One of them was audi-ology, which was led by the department chairperson. I really wanted to do well in this class and prove to myself that I could do the work.

I was the only guy in a class with thirty-five women. I always sat in the front so I wouldn't be distracted. I had my mini tape recorder with me to tape all of the classes. After class, I went home and transcribed all of the notes into my binder. I studied every day and memorized every word my pro-fessor said. I was memorizing ten to twelve pages every week. When an exam approached, all I had to do was read through my notes. I was still studying close to twenty-five hours per week for my two classes. My first exam came up and I got one of the top five scores in the class, which surprised some, but not me. I knew that if I continued to work hard, to persevere, and to be encouraged by my classmates, I would do well.

My second course was Stuttering and Neurological Disorders, which was led by Dr. Steers. By now, I knew a lot more about him. I knew he wanted me to be successful in whatever I was going to do with my life. He was one of my biggest supporters. He had one very interesting assignment. He asked my classmates to stutter in public, but for me it was the opposite. The students who did it felt very scared and frightened by stuttering. One of them said, "Bill, kudos to you for dealing with your stutter." It made me feel good.

I still had difficulty taking notes. One of my classmates let me borrow her notes for the class. By now, I had several friends in my classes and we were there to support each other. I did well in both my classes. I got a B-plus in audiology and a B in the stuttering class.

I was down to my final semester, which meant I would have the opportunity to work with kids as an undergraduate therapist. At least that's what I thought was going to happen. To my surprise, the department chairperson let me know I wasn't going to do therapy. Even though I had made a lot of progress with my language challenges, they thought it was best that I didn't provide therapy. They were concerned that I wouldn't be able to think quickly enough to provide the right kind of treatment. In the beginning, I was upset because I had worked so hard for this. In the end, though, I trusted my professors and believed they had my best interests in mind. They made an exception for me. Instead, I took another hearing course. My classmates were also very understanding.

Besides being around my classmates, I spent another year at the rooming house with the friends I had made the previous year. I had a lot of fun, especially playing Tecmo Bowl with my housemates and friends. We played all the time.

I ended up getting a 3.7 overall GPA and a 2.9 GPA in my major for my final year of college. Not bad for nearly failing out of the major. What really made the difference was reaching out to my classmates, tutors, and professors, who were interested in contributing to my success and being part of my team.

What would have really made a difference for me in college is letting go of my paranoia and nervousness about stuttering. I had let the fear of it dictate what I did and when I did it. There were several women I was interested in dating and who seemed interested in getting to know me, but I was always too afraid to ask them out on a date. I was consumed by those thoughts. I let my negative thoughts about stuttering—and what I *thought* women were thinking of me—stop me from dating. To this day, the "what might have been" thoughts weigh more heavily on me than what actually happened. I wanted to join student organizations. I wanted to go to dances. I wanted to go out on dates like "normal people," but I always reverted back to the excuse "because I stutter." There were a lot of things I wanted to do that I didn't because of that excuse. If I had let go of my fear of stuttering, or at least taken it less seriously, my college experience would have been filled with a lot more fun. I wouldn't have been so reserved; I would have let loose more. That isn't to say I didn't have fun in college, because I did. I had fun hanging out with my housemates and going to parties with them, but I could have had so much more. I resented my older brother for saying stuttering was "no big deal," but now I wish I hadn't taken it so seriously.

I graduated from West Chester University on May 15, 1993. I sat next to my friend Shirley, who had become a great friend since she had introduced herself to me eighteen months earlier. We were both excited about graduating. When my name was called, I shook the president's hand and got my degree. As I was walking off stage, I screamed at the top of my lungs, "Yes! I did it!" It took me seven years to get my bachelor's degree, but I made it. I failed a lot, but I never gave up. My family was proud of me and I was proud of myself.

It was six years later, in 1999, that I was finally able to move on with my dad. I called him and we had a real talk for the first time in a long time. It truly felt as if a great weight had been lifted off my shoulders, and his, too. Now we had the opportunity to create a father-son relationship again, and we have. The twenty years since then have been free of the anger, hatred, and resentment that marked the previous years. We were both brave and loving enough to apologize, and forgive, in our own ways.

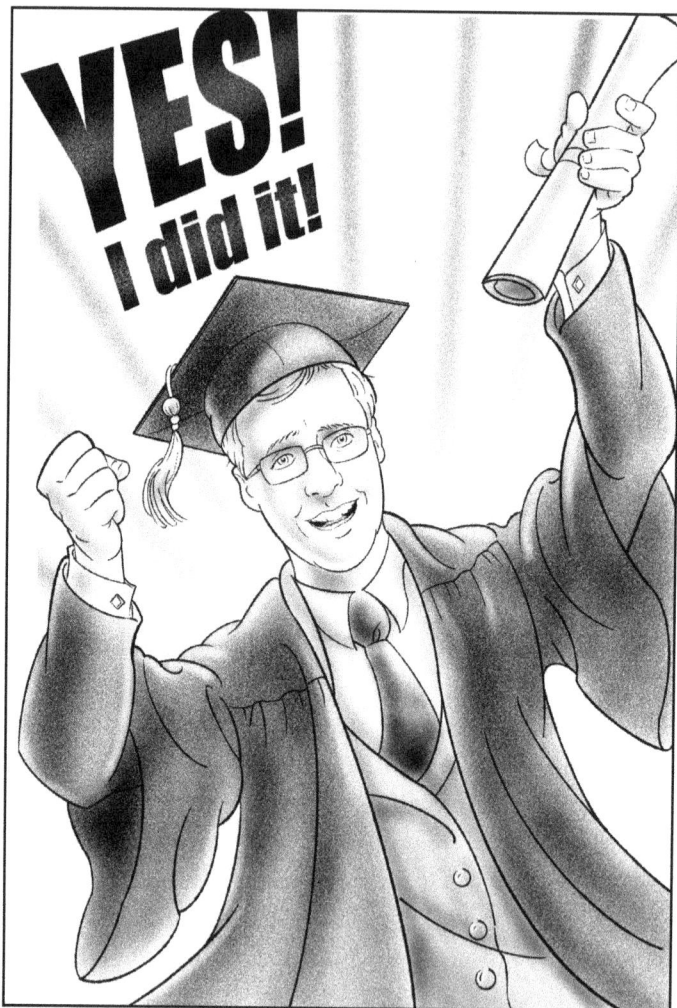

Writing this book opened up old wounds. And after being so honest about my childhood, I worried my dad might think that I defined him by it. For this reason, I called my dad again one evening and said even more than I did that day in 1999. I said, "Dad, I want you to know that I'm proud of what you have accomplished in your life. You were married for nearly thirty years and did your best to make it work. You got remarried to a wonderful woman who loved you dearly. You raised three boys and a stepdaughter and stepson. In 1990, you stopped drinking and have been sober ever since. You gave up cigarettes in 1996 and made a commitment to your health by walking and working out. You have always given me great advice. You're a great listener and you're always straight in your communication. You have been one of my biggest supporters, especially with my speaking career, and I really appreciate that."

I don't know what effect my words had on him, and that doesn't matter. We have enjoyed a lot of fun times together, meeting in New Jersey and visiting him in Myrtle Beach, going to dinner and riverboat gambling. I am glad I had the chance to see him and his wife Lisa as many times as I did because she passed away too young. Since then, I haven't seen my dad as much, but I call him regularly and have a lot of wonderful phone conversations with him.

My parents played a huge role in making me the person I am today. Though childhood had its challenges, I love and appreciate everything my parents provided for me. I learned a lot from the experience of being their son. My father taught me to stand up for myself. I could not expect people to stop teasing me if I let them think it was okay. My mother taught me what it meant to have someone in my corner who supported me.

As I got older and learned how to find a team of people who could provide me with support, together we let others know it was not okay to tease, torment, or laugh at me. I learned to be courageous in the face of obstacles and fear. I also learned to be resilient. I learned to persevere and never stop until I reached my goals: speaking fluently, doing well in school, and being part of the high school football team. I refused to let anyone define my limits. These characteristics have gotten me where I am now. I have overcome a severe stutter, a learning disability, and so many other challenges.

Aside from establishing a solid work ethic, my college experience taught me how important it is to have others support me in achieving my goals. Once I had set my goal of graduating college, I knew I had to step beyond my fear of stuttering and introduce myself to others. Not only did I excel and find fulfillment when I reached out to others, but contributing to my success also fulfilled them.

I spent the summer of 1993 at the Golden Slipper Camp. I had stayed in touch with Tim and my camper friend, Holly. I had familiarity going for me. I promised the director of the camp I would really be connected and fully involved with the campers. That year I wasn't with my friend Tim. I had two new counselors and I was with ten-year-old kids. I made sure to bring back-up batteries for my Fluency Master this time and it usually worked well. But I made a promise to myself that I was going to let it rip whether or not the Fluency Master worked, and I did. I got to know my campers really well. I got to hang out with Tim occasionally. He and I liked the same music. We both enjoyed Cat Stevens and John Denver. I led some of the activities even when I wasn't sure what to do. I just did it. I had fun. I made new friends. And every moment was made even more sweet by the knowledge that when camp was over, I wouldn't be coming back to do it again. It was time to move forward into the next chapter of my life.

In my professional career, as with college, the key to my success has been building a team to support me in my endeavors. I was bullied terribly by other kids, by my father, and mostly by myself, but I succeeded by letting go of my fear, taking risks, persevering, and having a team around me.

No matter how dark your reality seems, there are people in your life that really do care about you, some of whom you have yet to meet. So my advice to you is this: go create a team. Share your problems and fears with them. Reach out to the people who care about you and ask them to support you in achieving your goals. Take risks. The more people you have in your life, the more opportunities there are for growth and development. Get off the bench and get into the game. I grew stronger and more confident with every fear I faced. You can, too.

Conclusion

A question I get asked frequently is, "Bill, how did you overcome your stutter?"

Many years ago, I made a choice not to let the fear of stuttering stop me in my life. Up until 2003, I looked at myself as a victim of stuttering. Then, I decided to make a list of all the things I didn't even try to do because of my stutter.

That list, which included striking up conversations with people I didn't know and working at jobs in which my main responsibility was to speak with others, led to me becoming a bank teller.

Each interaction I had with a customer gave me the chance to face my fear of speaking with others. The more I did it the easier interacting with customers and coworkers became. I really enjoyed it. Within a year of working, I knew all the customers on a first-name basis.

One day, a friend called me and suggested I become a motivational speaker. He said, "Bill, you are one of the most inspiring people I know. I was just at a Les Brown speaker training and you need to go to the next one." The next challenge was upon me. It was no longer a wish. It was about to become a reality. There was just one hitch. He told me it was $1,000 for the training and another $1,000 for airfare, a hotel, and food. I didn't have the money, but one of the bank customers generously offered to pay for me to go.

Three days later I was in Orlando, Florida with the great

Les Brown and 75 aspiring speakers. At the training, I had to give a short talk. I was so nervous I stuttered on every word. In the end, people were inspired by my courage. I also had the opportunity to speak with Les Brown for a few minutes and take a picture with him. I left the training with enthusiasm and excitement. I was ready to get paid to do speaking events.

After a year of making cold calls, I finally booked my first paid speaking event for Monday, October 23, 2006. I spoke with 500 middle-school students. As you can imagine, I was very nervous. For the first 10 minutes of my talk, all the students laughed at me. It brought back a lot of painful memories, but I knew I had to push through. Eventually, my nervousness went away and I delivered the rest of my talk with enthusiasm. As I was leaving the auditorium, the students started chanting, "Bill! Bill! Bill! Bill!" That felt great.

A week later I got called to do 3 separate assemblies with 9th graders in Delaware at a charter school. For each assembly, the students laughed when I began to stutter. But this time, I said something to them about it. I said, "Whatever you see in me you see in yourselves. You are not laughing at me you are laughing at yourselves." With that you could hear a pin drop in the room.

I could have stopped when they laughed at me, but that would have made no difference. What made the biggest difference was THAT I believed in myself and trusted that I could deliver a great message. After that, I was hooked. I delivered several more talks locally over the next few years and each time students laughed at my stutter. But it no longer bothered me.

In the fall of 2009, I delivered a talk to 550 9th graders for 45 minutes. I didn't stutter. No one laughed at me. That became my new normal. I delivered inspiring talks to middle schools, high schools, and even colleges around the country.

To truly feel self-confident in my ability to book a college event, it took me 3 years of making phone calls. It wasn't easy.

At times it was frustrating, and it seemed every time I was close to getting a 'Yes' to speak at a college, it would turn into a 'No'. It took me 3,500 calls before I booked my first paid college event.

I know there are goals and dreams in your life you want to achieve. It is time for you to face your fears. Make a list of them. Tackle each one. Run toward your fears. It might not be easy, but the more you do it the easier it will get. You can do this. You can achieve your goals and dreams.

Afterword

I met Bill Deering for the first time over 35 years ago and I have always admired his perseverance and courage. After reading this book, I find myself even more impressed with Bill and what he has overcome. Frankly, I am humbled.

Bill was quite generous about the little things I did for him in high school; however, I was only one of a tight-knit group of caring and special friends. That whole group relied on and rallied around each other. There were also some incredible high-school coaches that provided a great deal of support. In this book, Bill appropriately emphasized the importance of building a team, and our group was just that.

I believe this book will provide people who struggle with stuttering, or some other form of disability, valuable life lessons told from the perspective of someone who has walked in their shoes, never given up, and who now shares his message with very large audiences.

Bill's story emphasizes so many important life lessons. Sadly, many of these lessons are ignored or forgotten by most people. All Bill sought while growing up was to be what others consider a normal kid. Tragically, very few of those around Bill were, in Bill's words, "brave souls willing to extend kindness." The overwhelming percentage of people Bill encountered were either unaware of how to react to his stuttering, weren't interested enough to react, or were just plain mean. This book should be mandatory for any teacher or coach who interacts with people who stutter.

Hopefully, it will provide reminders for all about how destructive bullying is and how important it is to show tolerance, acceptance, and love. Everyone goes through challenges. Sometimes it's obvious, while at other times, it's less noticeable to the outside world. Either way, extending kindness rarely takes much effort, but it can and does have a profound effect on the people it touches.

Maya Angelou's quote, "People will forget what you said, people will forget what you did, but people will never forget how you made them feel," is so relevant to the message of this book. It seems so simple, but many don't extend the minimal effort it takes to make someone else feel a little better, if only for a moment.

To this day, I remain in awe of Bill and his courage and discipline to overcome the struggle he wakes up to every single day. I feel thankful that, in a small way, my actions along with those of my friends helped Bill to get through such a difficult time.

I hope this book inspires everyone who reads it to remember how much a seemingly small act of kindness can make for another person. I also hope all who read this book look for ways to make others feel better, if only with the power of a quick smile.

Chris Bright

Acknowledgments

Dear Friends & Classmates,

I really appreciate all of you. Some of you I may not have know as well as others, but I do appreciate how respectful, caring, and loving you were with me. Thank you for saying "hello" to me in passing, for sitting with me at lunch and for the encouragement you showed me. Thank you to all the people I had a chance to be around on the football and track teams. Thank you to all the people I had a chance to be with in high school especially my last two years. The little things meant so much to me. The smiles, the hugs, and the conversations we had. Those are the things I will remember most about you.

I want to offer a special thanks to the people who I really connected with over the years. Though I didn't say very much, I did appreciate your patience in letting me get out my words even when it felt like forever to do so. You taught me perseverance, courage, teamwork, friendship, and love.

Thank you to the following people who were a contribution to me. They are:

Chris Bright – Thank you for introducing yourself to me at the summer training program for football in 1984. I appreciate you introducing me to all your friends. Thank you for running the last 200 meters with me around the track when I was ready to quit. Thank you for all the encouragement you gave me. You were a difference maker in my life. I love and appreciate you.

Steve D'Amico – You give it to me straight and I really appreciate it. You have been a great friend.

Doc Doyle – Thank you for always giving it to me straight. I appreciated all the sessions of progressive relaxation you did with me on your off time to help me with my stutter. Thank you.

Angie Ganser – You were a great teacher. I appreciate how kind and generous you were with me throughout my high school years.

Mike Herbert – You were like a father figure to me. You were there for me in the good and bad times. I certainly appreciate all the conversations we had regardless of the time of day. You were a great mentor and friend. I miss you.

Anthony Holowsko – You were a good friend who listened to me even when it took me several minutes to say something. You took me out to dinner when I was finishing up speech therapy in the summer of 1987. It meant a lot to me.

Tom Hynes – You gave me great words of wisdom. You said, "Quality time over quantity time". That made a difference for me. Thank you.

Darin Lugat – You were one of the people I felt very comfortable speaking with even when it took me several minutes to say something.

John McGready – You have been a great friend for a long time. Thank you for being there for me.

Mary Messa – You always believed in me and accepted me for who I was.

Zane Moore – You were one of the first people I met at West Chester University. You put me at ease. You were easy to talk with about anything. We had some great laughs and fun together. Thank you.

Nick Perna – You made indoor track fun with your playful personality. You were a kind and compassionate friend.

Dave Richards – You took me aside in March of 1985 and

told me I needed to lose weight to improve in the shot put and discus. You supported and encouraged me through the process. Thank you.

Rich Rogers – Thank you for being a good friend and for listening to me.

Ron Rotelli – You put me at ease. I loved when you finished my sentences for me. That certainly made it a lot easier. You had a great sense of humor. You were one of my closest friends and I miss you.

Heather Shafter – I am so glad we met in the summer of 1992. You have been one of my closest friends for a long time. Thank you, for all the editing you did for my book. You are a very talented and creative writer. You are easy to talk with and you are a lot of fun to hang with. Thank you for being a great friend.

Cheryl Shiley – Thank you for introducing yourself in the fall of 1991. I appreciate you helping and encouraging me through communication disorders. You were a great friend.

Dave Sowers – You listened to me and that meant a lot.

Milt Stewart – You give great advice and you are always straight with me. I appreciate that.

Joe Stigora – You were a great professor, mentor, and friend. I appreciate you introducing me to the Fluency Master and for the encouragement you have given me throughout the years.

Tim Stokes – You were one of the first people who introduced yourself to me when I came to the football summer training program. When I stuttered severely it was no big deal to you. You accepted me. You inspired me by your work ethic, courage, and determination.

Lou Wade – You were the first coach who pushed me to play aggressive and box out. You also gave me the nickname of Big' Un which I really loved and still do to this day.

Dave White – You encouraged me to stick with speech therapy when I wanted to quit. I loved your upbeat personality. I miss you.

Bill Wilson – I loved being around you for your grit and determination and your love for your friends and family.

Alayne Bianco – Your kindness meant a lot to me.

Resources

The Arc

The Arc protects the human rights of people with disabilities and their families. I had an opportunity several years ago to be the opening speaker at one of its events.

https://www.thearc.org

Association on Higher Education and Disability (AHEAD)

AHEAD is a professional membership association that provides support to students with disabilities in higher education. This association holds international conferences and webinars that attract disability staff from colleges and universities around the US and beyond.

https://www.ahead.org

BetterHelp

BetterHelp offers suggestions regarding how you may find free classes through community agencies and organizations for anger management. It also offers convenient online therapy with over 20,000 licensed therapists. You can text, email, or video chat with your therapist from the comfort of your home or anywhere else you have Internet access. The platform's articles are informative, thorough, and beneficial to those seeking solutions to their challenges.

https://www.betterhelp.com

Different & Able

Different & Able is a community of people who work to inspire and support each other. The website offers inspirational stories about people who haven't been limited by their disability and are making a difference in the world.

https://www.differentandable.org

Easter Seals

Easter Seals has supported people with disabilities, veterans, seniors, and their families for more than 100 years. Its mission is to provide exceptional services to ensure all people have equal opportunities to live, learn, work, and play in their communities.

easterseals.com

National Association of People Against Bullying (NAPAB)

NAPAB advocates for victims of bullying. They offer services such as therapy, martial arts, and private investigations. I like their "Cool 2 Be Kind" club, which has over 100 locations in the United States.

www.napab.org

National Stuttering Association (NSA)

NSA works to change the lives of people who stutter. They offer resources, events, and support to adults and teens. I attended the **NSA Annual Conference** one year when it was held in Arizona. It was an enriching opportunity and everyone was friendly and accommodating.

https://westutter.org, #westutter, 1-800-westutter

Stop Bullying

Stop Bullying is a government agency dedicated to the eradication of all bullying, including cyber bullying. They provide resources to recognize and prevent bullying. They have an extensive online training center tailored to bulky prevention stakeholders.

stopbullying.gov

Stuttering Association for the Young (SAY)

SAY is dedicated to supporting young people who stutter and the people in their lives. They offer programs such as summer camps, speech therapy, and creative arts programming to build the confidence and communication skills necessary for a child to thrive. This is a very cool organization for kids who stutter.

www.say.org

Stuttering Foundation

Stuttering Foundation offers free online resources, services, and support to people that stutter and their families. The foundation also serves as a resource for researchers committed to understanding the causes of stuttering.

https://www.stutteringhelp.org

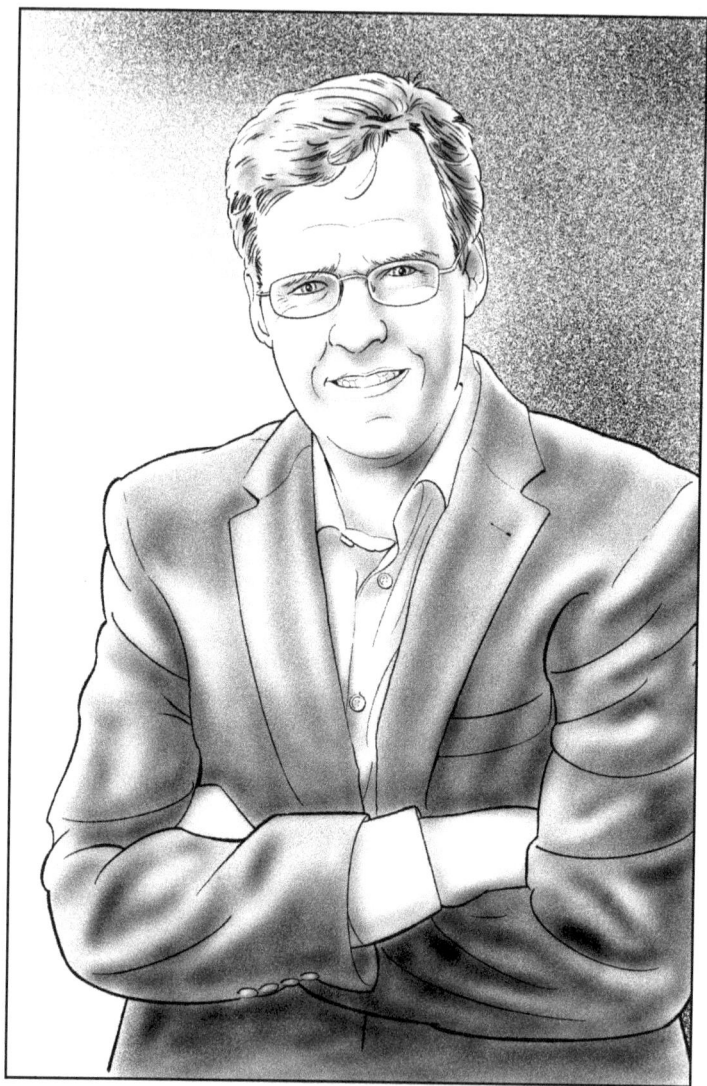

About the Author

Bill Deering is a Motivational Speaker committed to making a difference for others. He graduated from West Chester University of Pennsylvania in 1993 with a Bachelor's degree in Communication Disorders.

The career choice of motivational speaker was not an obvious one. When Bill was in middle school, he was often picked on for his stuttering. By the end of his sophomore year in high school, Bill had no friends, was 55 pounds overweight, and failing most of his classes.

The summer before his junior year, Bill made the life-changing decision to go out for the football team. Everything changed after that. By the time he graduated, Bill had the admiration of his classmates and teachers. However, Bill's stutter continued to plague him well into his twenties. One day, someone suggested that his stutter could be an advantage, and it changed his life. Bill stopped living as a victim of stuttering and began living from a place of power and freedom. He discovered that his fear of stuttering didn't have to stop him.

Bill has tackled each new challenge in his life – middle school, high school, college, and a career as a motivational speaker – with a passion and perseverance that inspires all who know him. Bill's keynotes have been described as "empowering," "heartening," and "inspiring." Since completing speaker training with Les Brown in 2005, he has delivered his message of courage, power, and passion to over 30,000 people. Bill was inducted into his high school hall of fame in 2022.

Follow Bill Deering:

Facebook:	https://www.facebook.com/bill.deering.50
LinkedIn:	https://linkedin.com/in/bill-deering-5380893
Twitter:	@bdspeaksout
Website:	https://www.billdeering.net

www.ingramcontent.com/pod-product-compliance
Lightning Source LLC
Chambersburg PA
CBHW071028280326
41935CB00011B/1495